Musculoskeletal Ultrasound Teaching Files

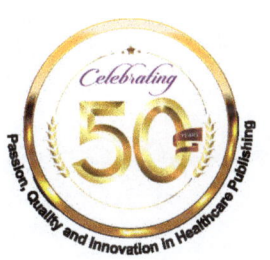

Musculoskeletal Ultrasound Teaching Files

Bipin R Shah
MD DMRD DMRE
Director
Eclat Polyclinic, Mumbai
Gray Scale Imaging, Mumbai
Lifescan Imaging
Mumbai, Maharashtra, India

Ankit B Shah
DNB MD Pg Dip MSK Ultrasound (UCAM Spain)
Consultant Radiologist
Eclat Polyclinic, Mumbai
Gray Scale Imaging
Mumbai, Maharashtra, India

Foreword
Nidhi Bhatnagar

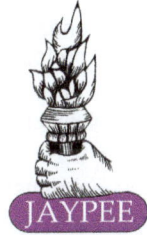

JAYPEE BROTHERS MEDICAL PUBLISHERS
The Health Sciences Publisher
New Delhi | London | Panama

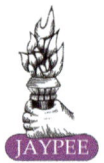
Jaypee Brothers Medical Publishers (P) Ltd

Headquarters

Jaypee Brothers Medical Publishers (P) Ltd
4838/24, Ansari Road, Daryaganj
New Delhi 110 002, India
Phone: +91-11-43574357
Fax: +91-11-43574314
Email: jaypee@jaypeebrothers.com

Overseas Offices

J.P. Medical Ltd
83 Victoria Street, London
SW1H 0HW (UK)
Phone: +44 20 3170 8910
Fax: +44 (0)20 3008 6180
Email: info@jpmedpub.com

Jaypee Brothers Medical Publishers (P) Ltd
Bhotahity, Kathmandu, Nepal
Phone: +977-9741283608
Email: kathmandu@jaypeebrothers.com

Jaypee-Highlights Medical Publishers Inc
City of Knowledge, Bld. 235, 2nd Floor
Clayton, Panama City, Panama
Phone: +1 507-301-0496
Fax: +1 507-301-0499
Email: cservice@jphmedical.com

Website: www.jaypeebrothers.com
Website: www.jaypeedigital.com

© 2019, Jaypee Brothers Medical Publishers

The views and opinions expressed in this book are solely those of the original contributor(s)/author(s) and do not necessarily represent those of editor(s) of the book.

All rights reserved. No part of this publication may be reproduced, stored or transmitted in any form or by any means, electronic, mechanical, photocopying, recording or otherwise, without the prior permission in writing of the publishers.

All brand names and product names used in this book are trade names, service marks, trademarks or registered trademarks of their respective owners. The publisher is not associated with any product or vendor mentioned in this book.

Medical knowledge and practice change constantly. This book is designed to provide accurate, authoritative information about the subject matter in question. However, readers are advised to check the most current information available on procedures included and check information from the manufacturer of each product to be administered, to verify the recommended dose, formula, method and duration of administration, adverse effects and contraindications. It is the responsibility of the practitioner to take all appropriate safety precautions. Neither the publisher nor the author(s)/editor(s) assume any liability for any injury and/ or damage to persons or property arising from or related to use of material in this book.

This book is sold on the understanding that the publisher is not engaged in providing professional medical services. If such advice or services are required, the services of a competent medical professional should be sought.

Every effort has been made where necessary to contact holders of copyright to obtain permission to reproduce copyright material. If any have been inadvertently overlooked, the publisher will be pleased to make the necessary arrangements at the first opportunity. The **CD/DVD-ROM** (if any) provided in the sealed envelope with this book is complimentary and free of cost. **Not meant for sale.**

Inquiries for bulk sales may be solicited at: jaypee@jaypeebrothers.com

Musculoskeletal Ultrasound Teaching Files

First Edition: **2019**

ISBN 978-93-5270-683-9

Dedicated to
My lovely wife Saroj.

Dad, Mom, Aditi, Vedant, Prachi and my Teachers.

Bipin R Shah

Ankit B Shah

FOREWORD

My introduction to Dr Bipin R Shah is so unique, it makes you believe in destiny all over again. I had submitted a paper in Musculoskeletal Ultrasound on Callus evaluation for an International Conference in 2013. Dr Marnix Vanholsbeeck was the Scientific co-ordinator with Dr Tony Bouffard. Dr Bipin R Shah was a well-known Musculoskeletal Specialist and both these world authorities had been great friends of his for many a years. So naturally they approached him for a feedback on my work and that was the turning point for me and musculoskeletal ultrasound in India. I met him for the first time in presence of Dr Bouffard in Agra in 2014 and his humble, unpretentious, simple demeanour floored me so very completely.

My introduction to Ankit B Shah and that they were father-son duo, came much later. The brilliance of father could be seen transcending the next generation in a most blessed manner. The vision they hold has been very effectively translated in this work called *Musculoskeletal Ultrasound Teaching Files* which is the second book they have co-authored. They have authored first book on *Ultrasound of Shoulder* which is a perfect reminder of the deep faith they both hold in the useful application of musculoskeletal ultrasound in clinical practice.

Although, the emphasis of this work in the second book is on musculoskeletal ultrasound, it contains much more that will be of interest to those outside the field of radiology, indeed to anyone having a fascination with the world of diagnostics. It describes the related anatomy, sonoanatomy along with the sonopathology findings, differential diagnosis and a discussion which answers all the small questions and why is that may arise through the course of reading through the case history. The authors have selected well over 82 cases with nearly all common complaints afflicting muscles, bones, joints, soft tissues, tendons and ligaments with which a patient may walk into the clinic for diagnosis and treatment. Although, these cases may represent just a sample in the spectrum of related pathologies, they amply illustrate the importance of ultrasound as an important diagnostic tool in evaluating musculoskeletal system complaints, as also raising the bar in patient care. The case series are a celebration of how ultrasound has evolved to a position of awe and credibility in today's highly specialized world dominated by magnetic resonance imaging (MRI) and computed tomographs (CTs).

It is all here, honest expressions, serious purpose, clarity of thoughts and strength of conviction in demonstrating the ultrasound signs with high sensitivity and specificity in diagnosing musculoskeletal system-related pathologies through simple yet dynamic modality like ultrasound, literally rehabilitating this tool, to reclaim the dignity of sonologist from the self-proclaimed gatekeepers who nearly for a decade or more wield the medical world to indict the 'Inferiority' of others and confirm 'superiority' of themselves, returning it to those who toiled at a labor of 'ultrasound' love because of that burning passion and belief in them.

There is no doubt that for the Drs Bipin R Shah and Ankit B Shah, writing this book was a labor of love.

I think that Drs Bipin R Shah and Ankit B Shah, the inspiring father-son team can be confident that there will be many a grateful readers who will benefit from the broad-based overview of pathologies that can be diagnosed through musculoskeletal ultrasound having well-defined structured approach laid out in this book.

Nidhi Bhatnagar
MD (Radiodiagnosis) Pg Dip. MSK US (UCAM Spain)
Head
Department of Radiology
Mata Chanan Devi Hospital
New Delhi, India
Professor
UCAM, University of Murcia, Spain
Vice President
Musculoskeletal Ultrasound Society

PREFACE

After having authored *Step by Step Sonography of the Shoulder Joint* in the year 2010, we are now ready with *Musculoskeletal Ultrasound Teaching Files*. The concept of a general musculoskeletal ultrasound case-based book arose from our work experience in musculoskeletal ultrasound and close interaction with the orthopedic colleagues over the years. The objective of this book is to present the information that we, as authors, believe, is important for those learning musculoskeletal ultrasound and those who are practicing musculoskeletal ultrasound on a routine basis. The cases have been segregated based on the anatomic region involved. We have tried to cover the common pathologies encountered in day-to-day practice, leaving out the exceptional cases. Each case begins with a clinical history followed by ultrasound images with their description, diagnosis and relevant discussion pertaining to the case. In the case discussion, we have stressed on relative anatomy and certain points that need to be incorporated within the report, so that all the relevant information is conveyed to the referring orthopedic surgeons and physicians. We have made a conscious effort to refrain from commenting on controversial topics. We are sincerely hopeful that this book provides a pleasant experience to the readers and provides answers quickly and easily when they need them.

Bipin R Shah
Ankit B Shah

ACKNOWLEDGMENTS

At the outset, I would like to thank Ankit, without whom this book would not have been possible.

I would like to thank my family for enduring our erratic working hours throughout the time this book was being written. I would sincerely like to thank my staff at Eclat Polyclinic and Gray Scale Imaging for compilation of images and helping us draft the manuscript.

Bipin R Shah

I will begin with a big thank to my dad Dr Bipin R Shah, a pioneer in musculoskeletal ultrasound in India. He is solely responsible for kindling my interest in musculoskeletal ultrasound. He has been my source of inspiration and guiding force.

I am indebted to my mom, my wife Aditi and my sister Prachi for their never-ending support. I am grateful to all my colleagues from the orthopedic fraternity who have bestowed their faith in me and have added to my understanding of musculoskeletal pathologies.

A big shout out to Dr Nidhi Bhatnagar whom I really can't thank enough. She has always been a pillar of strength for me and someone I have always looked up to.

A special thanks to my buddies Shriji, Manish, Babu, Rishi, Amol, Shraddha, Ankit and Swarup.

I would like to thank Shri Jitendar P Vij (Group Chairman), Mr Ankit Vij (Managing Director), Ms Chetna Malhotra Vohra (Associate Director–Content Strategy), Ms Madhuri Aggarwal (Development Editor), and all the staff of M/s Jaypee Brothers Medical Publishers (P) Ltd, New Delhi, India, for their efforts and input enabling timely publication of the book.

So that I do not leave anybody out, I would like to sincerely thank everyone who has directly or indirectly contributed while writing the book.

Ankit B Shah

CONTENTS

CASES

1. Subacromial Impingement of the Rotator Cuff — 1
2. Partial-thickness Articular Surface Tear of the Rotator Cuff — 4
3. Full-thickness Tear of the Rotator Cuff — 7
4. Postoperative Retear of the Supraspinatus Tendon — 10
5. Calcific Tendinosis of the Rotator Cuff — 12
6. Subacromial-subdeltoid Bursal Inflammation — 15
7. Tear of the Subscapularis Tendon — 18
8. Tear of the Long Head of Biceps — 20
9. Tenosynovitis of the Biceps Tendon Sheath — 24
10. Adhesive Capsulitis of Shoulder — 25
11. Paralabral Cyst with Suprascapular Nerve Entrapment — 29
12. Acromioclavicular Joint Dislocation — 32
13. Traumatic Fat Necrosis — 34
14. Radial and Ulnar Nerve Injury — 36
15. Stretch Injury of the Radial Nerve — 39
16. Intramuscular Cysticercosis of the Triceps Muscle Belly — 41
17. Ulnar Nerve Neuritis — 43
18. Olecranon Bursitis — 44
19. Bicipitoradial Bursitis — 46
20. Tennis Elbow — 48
21. Calcific Tendinosis Involving the Common Flexor Origin — 51
22. Subcutaneous Rheumatoid Nodule — 53
23. Chronic Partial-thickness Tear of the Triceps Muscle — 55
24. Osseous Avulsion Injury of Triceps Tendon — 57
25. Distal Biceps Tendon Tear — 59
26. Partial-thickness Tear of the Ulnar Collateral Ligament of the Elbow — 60
27. Myositis Ossificans — 61
28. Volar Wrist Ganglion — 63
29. Carpal Tunnel Syndrome — 65
30. Fibrolipomatous Hamartoma of the Median Nerve — 68

31.	Peripheral Nerve Sheath Tumor of the Median Nerve	71
32.	Tenosynovitis of the Flexor Tendon Sheath at the Wrist Joint	73
33.	De Quervain's Tenosynovitis	74
34.	Attritional Tear of Extensor Tendon at the Wrist due to Chronic Impingement	77
35.	Inflammatory Tenosynovitis of Extensor Compartment IV Tendon Sheath at the Wrist Joint	78
36.	Epidermal Inclusion Cyst	81
37.	Trigger Finger	83
38.	Trigger Thumb	85
39.	Crystal Deposition Disease	86
40.	Ganglion Arising from the A2 Pulley	88
41.	Nodular Thickening of the A2 Pulley in a Known Case of Rheumatoid Arthritis	89
42.	Inflammatory Synovitis Involving the Metacarpophalangeal Joint	90
43.	Tenosynovitis with Tendinosis of the Flexor Tendons of the Finger due to a Retained Foreign Body	94
44.	Traumatic Full-thickness Tear of Flexor Digitorum Profundus Tendon	96
45.	Traumatic Full-thickness Tear of Extensor Pollicis Longus Tendon	97
46.	Giant-cell Tumor of Flexor-tendon Sheath of a Finger	98
47.	Giant-cell Tumor of Extensor Tendon of Finger	99
48.	Subungual Glomus Tumor	101
49.	Glomus Tumor	103
50.	Avulsion Injury of Ulnar Collateral Ligament Injury of Thumb	104
51.	Acute Partial-thickness Tear of the Adductor Muscles	106
52.	Greater Trochanteric Bursitis	108
53.	Partial-thickness Tear of Gluteus Medius Tendon	110
54.	High-grade Partial Thickness Hamstring Tear with Hematoma	113
55.	Partial-thickness Tear of the Rectus Femoris with Hematoma	116
56.	Acute Synovitis of the Right Hip	118
57.	Prepatellar Bursitis	119
58.	Superficial Infrapatellar Bursitis	122
59.	Sessile Exostosis	124
60.	Jumper's Knee	126
61.	Full-thickness Tear of the Patellar Tendon	128
62.	Full-thickness Tear of the Quadriceps Tendon	130
63.	Effusion in the Suprapatellar Recess	132
64.	Effusion in the Suprapatellar Recess with Lipoma Arborescens	134
65.	Baker's Cyst with Synovitis	135

66.	Baker's Cyst	137
67.	Tennis Leg	138
68.	Herniation of the Tibialis Anterior Muscle	140
69.	Morel-Lavallée Lesion	142
70.	Tendinosis of the Achilles Tendon with an Interstitial Tear	144
71.	Chronic Partial-thickness Tear of the Achilles Tendon	147
72.	Full-thickness Tear of Achilles Tendon	149
73.	Insertional Calcific Tendinosis of Achilles Tendon	151
74.	Retrocalcaneal Bursitis	152
75.	Haglund's Syndrome	153
76.	Tear of the Anterior Talofibular Ligament	154
77.	Chronic Tophaceous Gout	156
78.	Interstitial Tear of the Tibialis Posterior Tendon with Tenosynovitis	159
79.	Interstitial Tear of Peroneus Brevis Tendon	162
80.	Foreign Body Granuloma	164
81.	Pyomyositis	165
82.	Plantar Fasciitis	166

Index   *169*

Case 1

Subacromial Impingement of the Rotator Cuff

■ CLINICAL HISTORY

A 40-year-old male presented with intermittent pain in the left shoulder during mid-range of shoulder abduction, since 2 months.

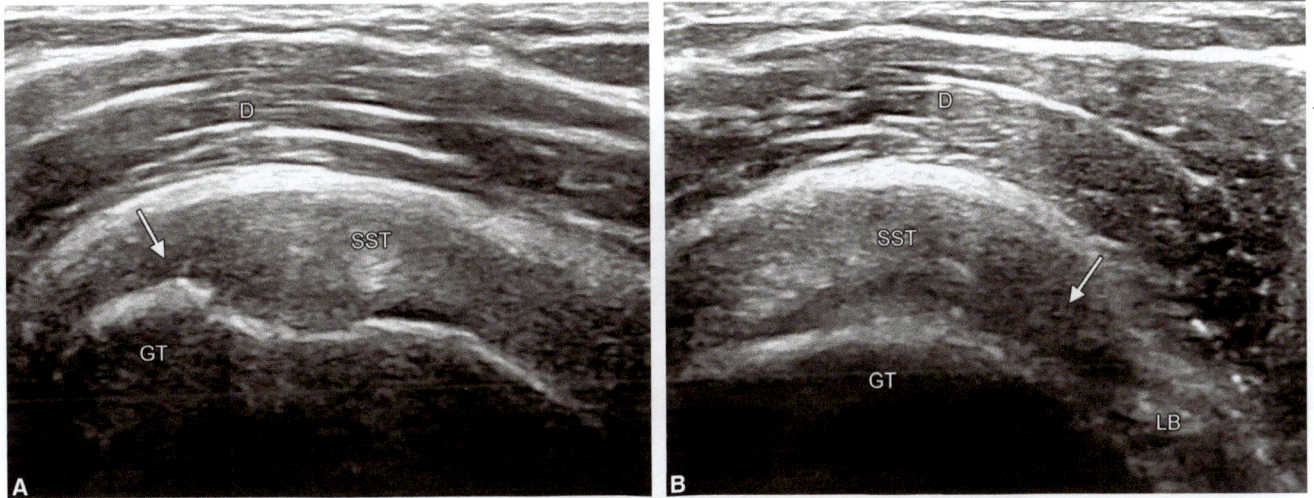

Figs. 1A and B: (A) Long-axis image shows an area of focal tendinosis (arrow) involving deep fibers of supraspinatus tendon (SST). There is no discontinuity of the fibers; and (B) Transverse image of the SST shows tendinosis (arrow) involving the anterior edge of the tendon immediately posterior to the long head of biceps (LB). (D: deltoid muscle; GT: greater tuberosity)

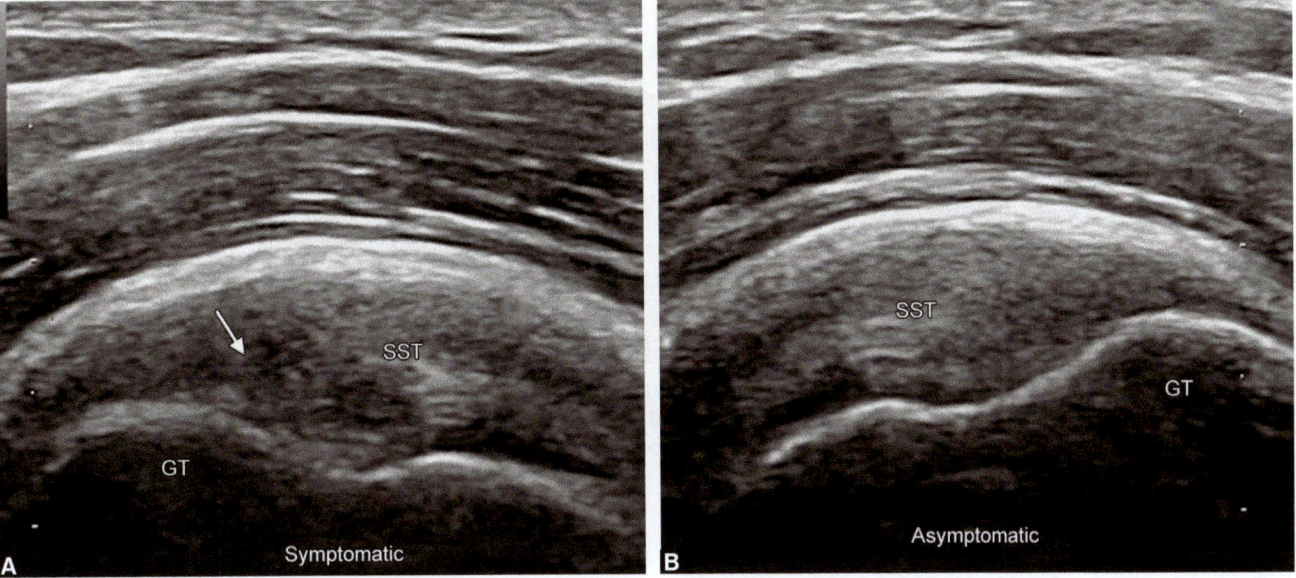

Figs. 2A and B: Comparison of long-axis images of the contralateral supraspinatus tendon (SST) makes the focal tendinosis (arrow) more obvious. (GT: greater tuberosity)

DIAGNOSIS

Focal tendinosis involving the supraspinatus tendon (subacromial impingement) (Figs. 1 and 2).

DISCUSSION

- The coracoacromial arch is a fibro-osseous tunnel formed by the acromion, acromioclavicular joint, coracoacromial ligament, coracoid, and the humeral head (Fig. 3).
- Any pathology affecting the coracoacromial arch can result in shoulder impingement. The pathology may compress the rotator-cuff tendon or the subacromial-subdeltoid (SASD) bursa against the coracoacromial arch or interrupt the smooth gliding of the rotator-cuff tendons passing below the coracoacromial arch.[1]
- Shoulder impingement is most often a clinical diagnosis.
- *Ultrasound (US) findings in shoulder impingement*:
    - Normal tendon
    - Tendinosis
    - Thickened SASD bursa/SASD bursal effusion
    - Spurs along the lateral margin of the acromion
    - Enthesopathic changes along the greater tuberosity
    - Coracoacromial ligament thickening.
- Tendinosis of the supraspinatus tendon may be focal or diffuse.

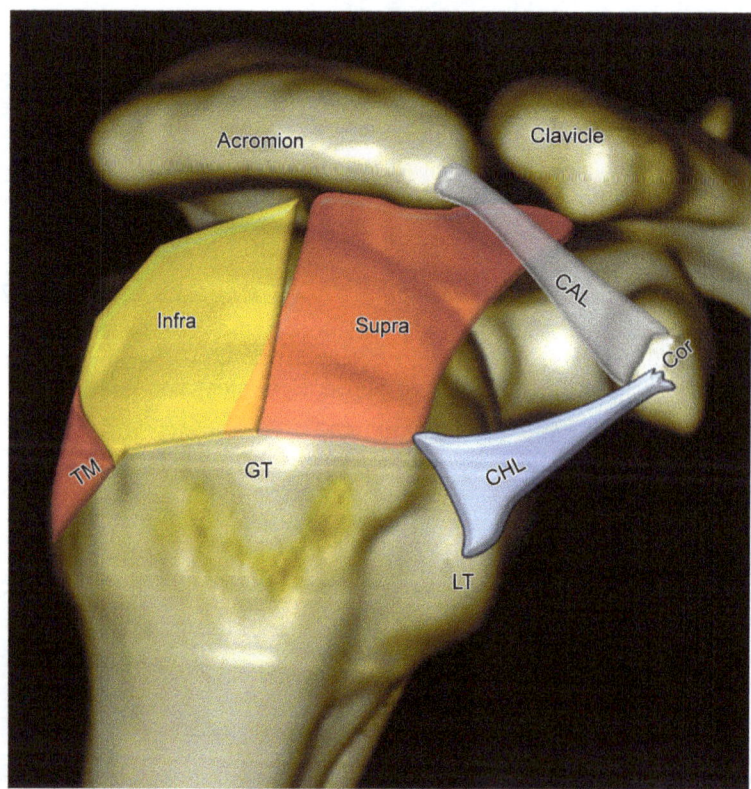

Fig. 3: Coracoacromial arch is a fibro-osseous tunnel formed by the acromion, coracoid (cor), the coracoacromial ligament (CAL), and the humeral head. The supraspinatus (supra), infraspinatus (infra), and the teres minor (TM) tendons pass below the coracoacromial arch. (CHL: coracohumeral ligament; GT: greater tuberosity; LT: lesser tuberosity)

- *Dynamic US signs of shoulder impingement:*
    - Bunching of the SA bursa against the lateral margin of the acromion.
    - Bunching of the supraspinatus tendon against the coracoacromial arch.
    - Incomplete sliding of the rotator-cuff tendon below the acromion during active movement.
    - Bulging of the coracoacromial ligament.[2]
- In adhesive capsulitis, incomplete sliding of the rotator-cuff below the acromion is seen during active as well as passive movements.
- A normal US scan does not rule out clinical shoulder impingement.[3]

REFERENCES

1. Bigliani LU, Levine WN. Subacromial impingement syndrome. J Bone Joint Surg Am. 1997;79:1854-68.
2. Wang YC, Wang HK, Chen WS, et al. Dynamic visualization of the coracoacromial ligament by ultrasound. J Ultrasound Med Biol. 2009;35:1242-8.
3. Awerbuch MS. The clinical utility of ultrasonography for rotator cuff disease, shoulder impingement syndrome and subacromial bursitis. Med J Aust. 2008;188:50-3.

CASE 2

Partial-thickness Articular Surface Tear of the Rotator Cuff

■ CLINICAL HISTORY

A 58-year-old lady presented with chronic left shoulder pain since 8 months. She is a known case of diabetes mellitus since 16 years.

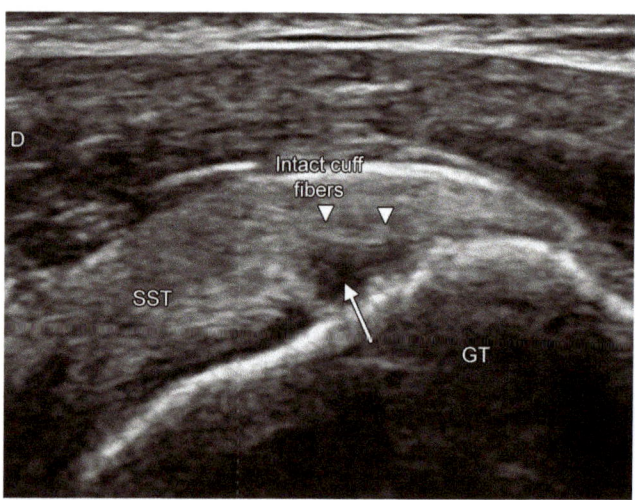 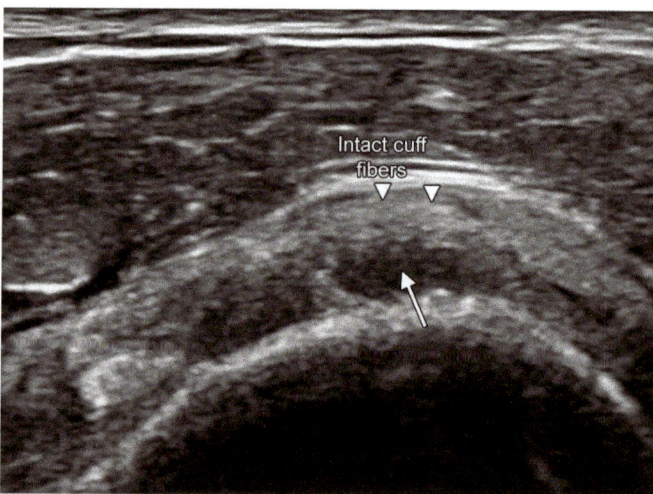

Fig. 1: Long-axis image shows a defect (arrow) involving articular surface fibers of the supraspinatus tendon (SST) along its footprint. The tear does not reach till the bursal surface—suggesting an articular surface tear. (D: deltoid muscle; GT: greater tuberosity)

Fig. 2: Transverse image shows the partial-thickness tear (arrow) to be involving posterior fibers of the supraspinatus tendon (SST) and the composite tendon.

■ DIAGNOSIS

Partial-thickness articular surface tear of the supraspinatus tendon (Figs. 1 and 2).

■ DISCUSSION

- The rotator cuff consists of subscapularis, supraspinatus, infraspinatus, and teres minor tendons and their muscle bellies. The muscles originate from the scapula and extend laterally, where their tendons blend imperceptibly to form a common tendon known as the rotator cuff. Except the subscapularis tendon which inserts over the lesser tuberosity, rest of the tendons insert over the greater tuberosity.
- Cuff tears may be either traumatic or degenerative. Degenerative tears are more commonly encountered than traumatic tears. Commonly proposed etiology for degenerative cuff tears are chronic microtrauma,[1] oxidative stress,[2] and suboptimal cuff vascularity.[3]

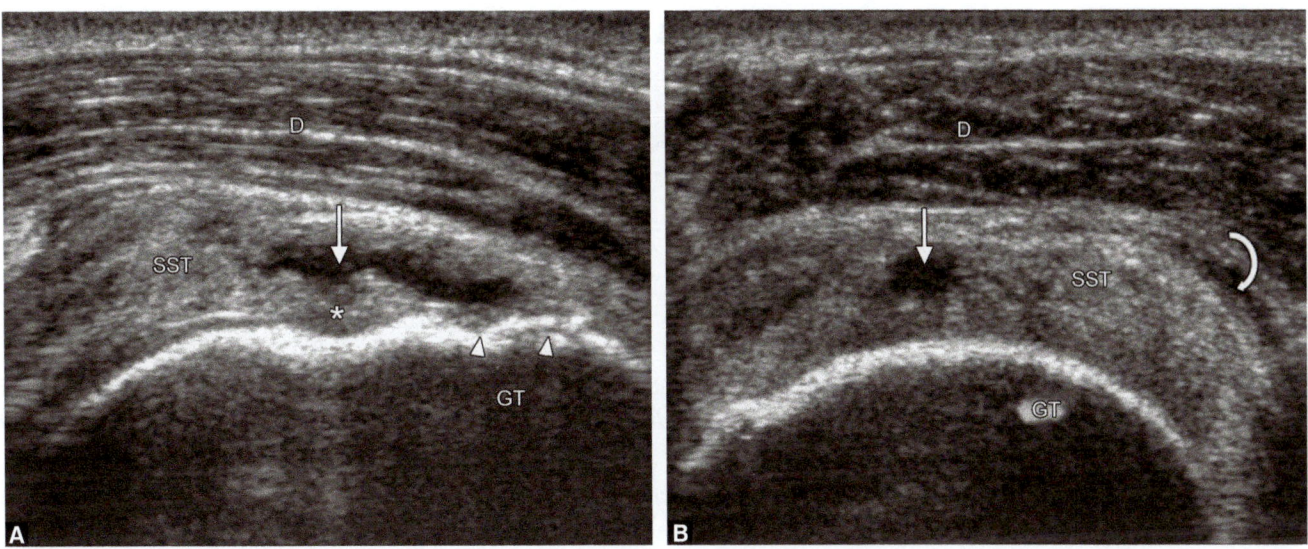

Figs. 3A and B: (A) Long-axis image shows discontinuity of the supraspinatus tendon (SST) fibers, suggesting an intratendinous tear (arrow) along its footprint. The tear does not reach either the bursal or the articular surface of the tendon—suggesting an intrasubstance tear. The adjacent fibers appear heterogeneous and hypoechoic (*), suggesting underlying tendinosis. Note the cortical irregularity (arrowheads) along the greater tuberosity (GT); and (B) Transverse image shows the partial-thickness tear (arrow) to be involving posterior fibers of the SST. Mild anechoic fluid is seen in the subacromial-subdeltoid bursa (curved arrow). (D: deltoid muscle)

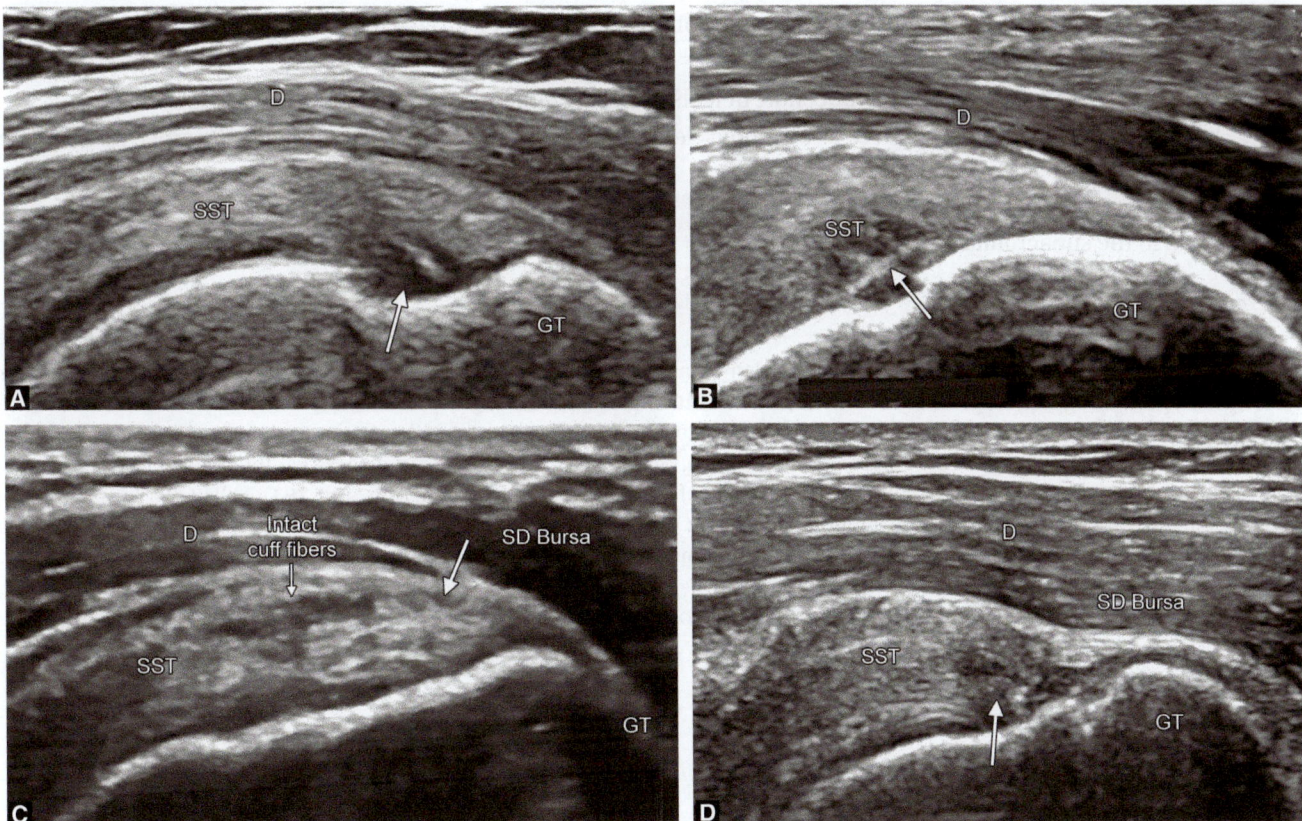

Figs. 4A to D: (A) Partial-thickness articular surface tear (white arrow); (B) Intrasubstance tear (white arrow); (C) Partial-thickness bursal surface tear (white arrow); and (D) Full-thickness tear (white arrow). (D: deltoid muscle; GT: greater tuberosity; SST: supraspinatus tendon; SD: subdeltoid)

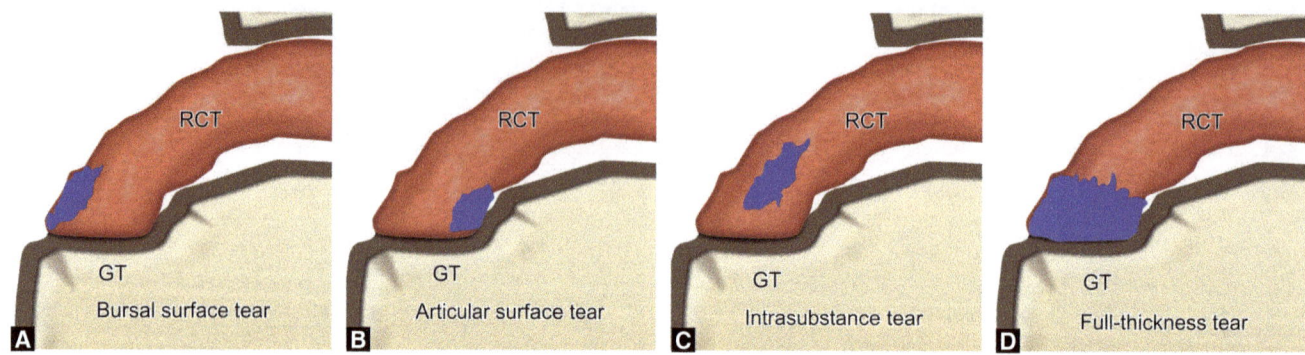

Figs. 5A to D: Types of tear depending on the site of involvement. (A) Bursal surface tear (partial thickness); (B) Articular surface tear (partial thickness); (C) Intrasubstance tear (partial thickness); and (D) Full-thickness tear. (GT: greater tuberosity; RCT: rotator cuff tendon)

- Degenerative tears are usually encountered in the anterior fibers of the supraspinatus tendon—approximately 7 mm posterior to the rotator interval.[4]
- Tears of the rotator cuff are broadly classified as partial-thickness (Figs. 3A and B) and full-thickness tears, depending on the location of the tear (Figs. 4A to D).[5]
- *Partial thickness tear (Figs. 5A to D) is classified as:*
  - Articular surface tear
  - Bursal surface tear
  - Intrasubstance tear.
- Articular surface tears are two to three times more common than bursal surface tears.[6]
- *Ultrasound findings in partial-thickness tears:*[7]
  - Well-defined focal anechoic or hypoechoic defects involving either the articular or bursal surface fibers.
    Intrasubstance tears are visualized as anechoic clefts bounded by intact articular and bursal surface fibers of the tendon.
  - Cortical irregularity over the greater tuberosity.
  - Fluid in the subacromial-subdeltoid bursa.

REFERENCES

1. Yamaguchi K, Ditsios K, Middleton WD, et al. The demographic and morphological features of rotator cuff disease. A comparison of asymptomatic and symptomatic shoulders. J Bone Joint Surg Am. 2006;88:1699-704.
2. Droge W. Oxidative stress and aging. Adv Exp Med Biol. 2003;543:191-200.
3. Lindblom K. On pathogenesis of ruptures of the tendon aponeurosis of the shoulder joint. Acta Radiol. 1939;20:563-77.
4. Codman EA. The pathology associated with the rupture of the supraspinatus tendon. Ann Surg. 1931;93:348-59.
5. Zlatkin MB. MRI of the Shoulder, 2nd edition. Lippincott: Williams and Wilkins; 2003.
6. Payne LZ, Altchek DW, Craig EV, et al. Arthroscopic treatment of partial rotator cuff tears in young athletes: a preliminary report. Am J Sports Med. 1997;25:299-305.
7. van Holsbeeck MT, Kolowich PA, Eyler WR, et al. US depiction of partial-thickness tear of the rotator cuff. Radiology. 1995;197:443-6.

CASE 3

Full-thickness Tear of the Rotator Cuff

■ CLINICAL HISTORY

A 43-year-old man presented with pain in the right shoulder with restricted overhead abduction since 2 months.

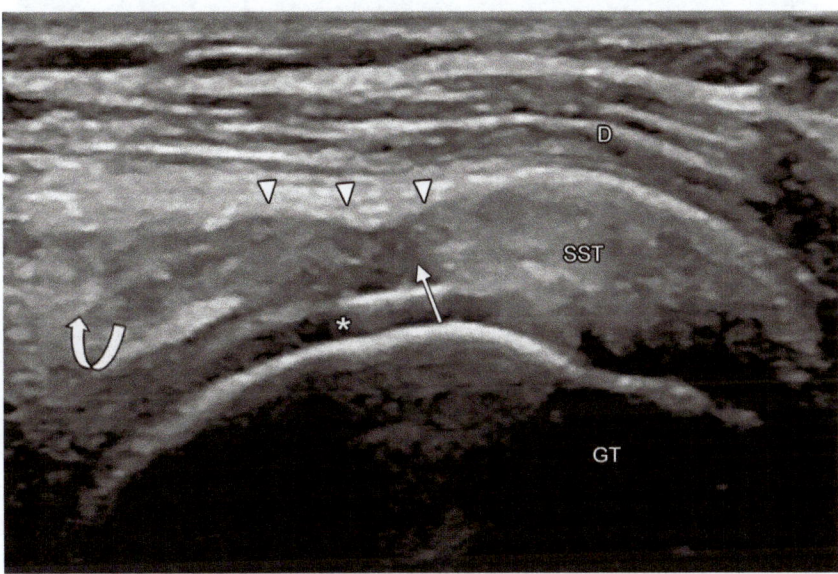

Fig. 1: Long-axis image shows discontinuity of the supraspinatus tendon (SST) fibers, suggesting a full-thickness tear (white arrow) in the critical zone of the tendon. The tear involves the bursal and the articular surfaces. The articular cartilage (*) covering the humeral head is well visualized (naked cartilage sign). The subacromial-subdeltoid bursa (arrowheads) sags into the defect resulting in a concave superior contour. Irregular edges (curved arrow) of the tear are seen retracted medially. (D: deltoid muscle; GT: greater tuberosity)

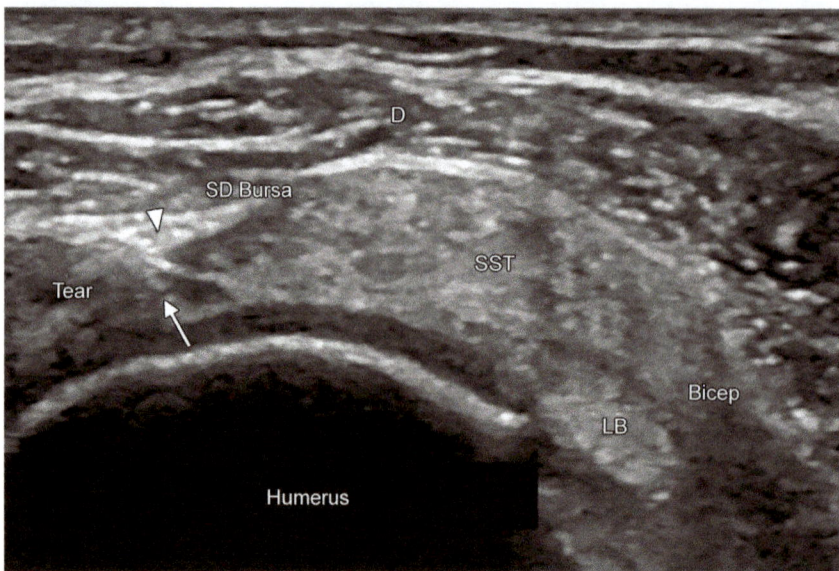

Fig. 2: Transverse image shows a full-thickness tear involving posterior fibers of the supraspinatus tendon (SST) and the composite tendon. The tear involves the bursal and the articular surfaces. The subacromial-subdeltoid bursa (arrowhead) sags into the defect resulting in a concave superior contour. (D: deltoid muscle; LB: long head of biceps; SD: subdeltoid)

■ DIAGNOSIS

Full-thickness tear of the supraspinatus tendon (Figs. 1 and 2).

■ DISCUSSION

- A full-thickness tear of the rotator cuff extends from articular till the bursal surface.
- 28–53% of partial-thickness tears progress to thickness tears.[1]

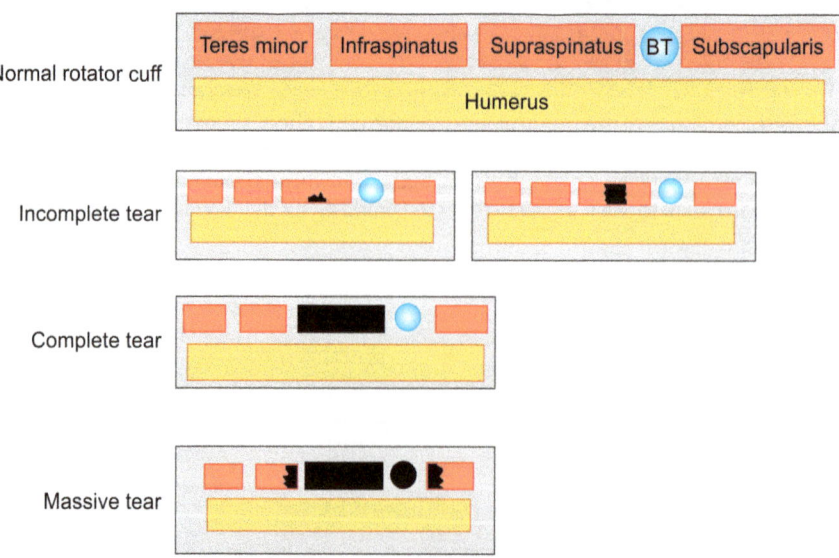

Fig. 3: Morphology of rotator cuff tears.

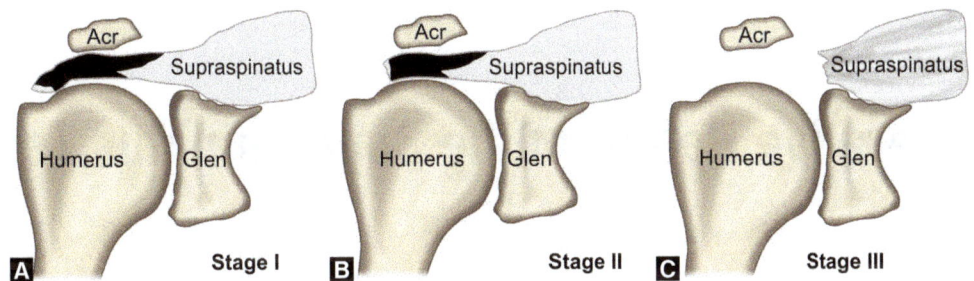

Figs. 4A to C: Stages of cuff tear retraction in the frontal plane. (A) Stage I—The torn edge is just above the greater tuberosity (GT); (B) Stage II—The torn edge lies over the humeral head; and (C) Stage III—The torn edge lies at the level or medial to the glenoid margin. (Glen: glenoid; Acr: acromion)

- *Ultrasound (US) findings in full-thickness tear*:
    - Intratendinous fluid-filled anechoic or hypoechoic defects.
    - "Double cortex" or "cartilage interface" sign wherein the uncovered cartilage covering the humeral head appears accentuated.
    - Focal depressions of the peribursal fat [subacromial-subdeltoid bursa] within the defect caused due to tendon tear (*sagging peribursal fat* sign).
    - Atrophy of the torn muscle.
    - Medial retraction of the torn edges.
    - Fatty infiltration of infraspinatus muscle is an indicated the possibility of a multitendon tear.[2]
- **Reporting checklist for US evaluation of a cuff tear:**
    - Partial or full-thickness tear.
    - *Location of the partial thickness tear*: Articular/bursal/intrasubstance.
    - Percentage of cuff thickness involved in partial thickness tear.
    - Distance of the full thickness tear from the biceps tendon (Fig. 3).[3]
    - Condition of the fibers adjacent to the torn margins.
    - Anteroposterior dimension of the tear.
    - Level of retraction of the edges (adjacent to the greater tuberosity/at humeral head/medial to the acromion) (Figs. 4A to C).[3]
    - Supraspinatus/infraspinatus muscle atrophy.[3]
    - Presence of cortical irregularity in over the greater tuberosity.
    - Subacromial (SA) bursa (effusion/synovial hypertrophy/presence of synovial vascularity on power Doppler).
    - Effusion in the biceps tendon sheath/tendinosis of the long head of biceps.
    - Acromioclavicular joint (synovial hypertrophy/marginal osteophytes/spurs along lateral margin of the acromion).

REFERENCES

1. Yamanaka K, Matsumoto T. The joint side tear of the rotator cuff. A follow-up study by arthrography. Clin Orthop Relat Res. 1994;304:68-73.
2. Melis B, Wall B, Walch G. Natural history of infraspinatus fatty infiltration in rotator cuff tears. J Shoulder Elbow Surg. 2010;19:757-63.
3. Arce G, Bak K, Bain G, et al. Management of disorders of the rotator cuff: proceedings of the ISAKOS Upper Extremity Committee Consensus Meeting. Arthroscopy. 2013;29:1840-50.

Case 4

Postoperative Retear of the Supraspinatus Tendon

■ CLINICAL HISTORY

A middle-aged man presented with persistent left shoulder pain during abduction of the arm. He was operated for a full-thickness tear of the rotator cuff 4 years ago.

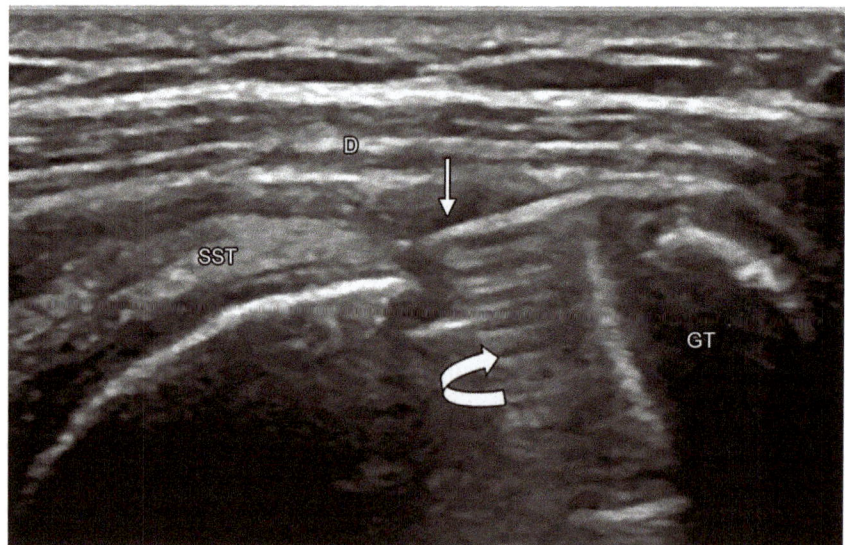

Fig. 1: Complete discontinuity of the supraspinatus tendon (SST) fibers suggests a recurrent tear (straight arrow). The anchor (curved arrow) is well embedded within the greater tuberosity (GT). (D: deltoid muscle)

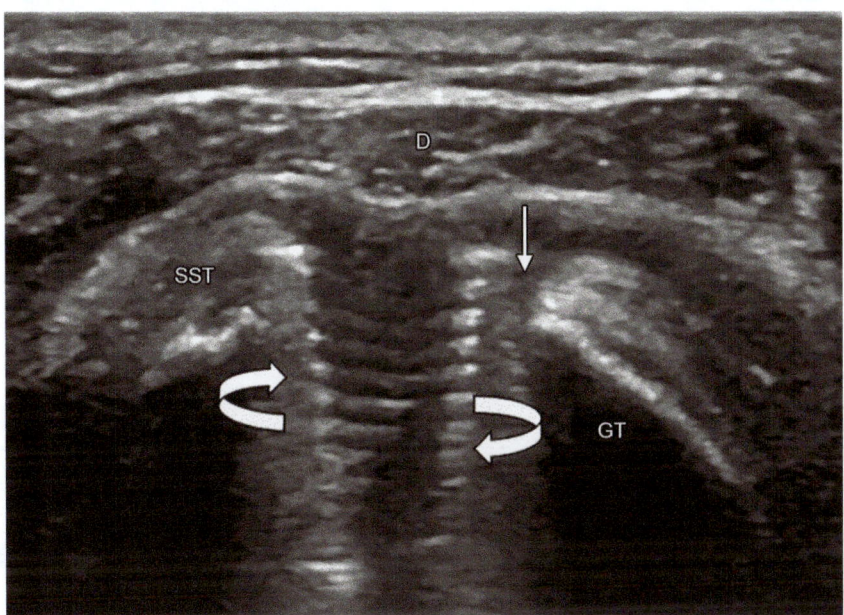

Fig. 2: Transverse images show the deltoid muscle (D) herniating within the defect caused by the recurrent tear (straight arrow) of the supraspinatus tendon (SST). The anchors are depicted by the curved arrows. (GT: greater tuberosity)

■ DIAGNOSIS

Full-thickness retear of the supraspinatus tendon.

■ DISCUSSION

- The incidence of cuff failure following a rotator-cuff repair ranges from 14% to 94%.[1]
- Absence of artifacts from the metallic implants and dynamic imaging make ultrasound (US) an ideal modality for evaluation of the postoperative cuff.
- Heterogeneous echotexture of the rotator cuff is a normal postoperative finding. This finding may persist for months to years after the surgery.
- Recurrent tears are diagnosed on US on the basis of partial- or full-thickness defects within the cuff at the site of tendon repair along the greater tuberosity (Figs. 1 and 2).

■ REFERENCE

1. Bishop J, Klepps S, Lo IK, et al. Cuff integrity after arthroscopic versus open rotator cuff repair: a prospective study. J Shoulder Elbow Surg. 2006;15:290-9.

CASE 5

Calcific Tendinosis of the Rotator Cuff

■ CLINICAL HISTORY

A 27-year-old lady presented with acute pain and stiffness in the right shoulder since morning. There is no history of trauma.

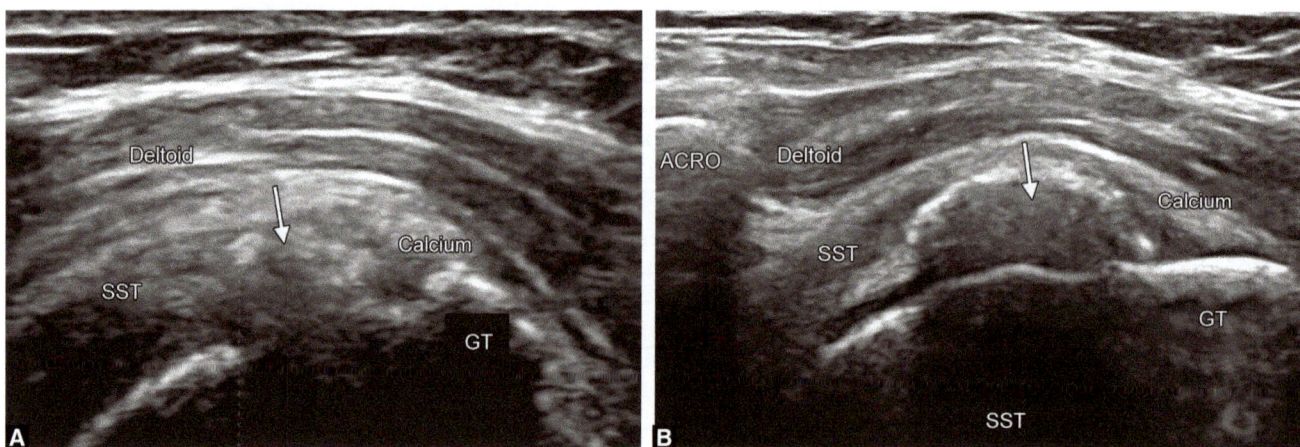

Figs. 1A and B: Calcification within the supraspinatus tendon (SST) is seen as nodular echogenic intratendinous foci (arrows) with varying degree of distal shadowing. (GT: greater tuberosity; ACRO: acromion)

■ DIAGNOSIS

Calcific tendinosis involving the supraspinatus and infraspinatus tendons with extrusion of calcium into the subacromial-subdeltoid (SASD) bursa.

■ DISCUSSION

- Calcific tendinosis of the rotator cuff is characterized by intratendinous deposition of calcium hydroxyapatite. This is a self-limiting condition.
- The incidence of calcific tendinosis in healthy adult shoulders ranges from 2.5% to 7.5%.[1]
- The commonly affected tendons are: supraspinatus (80%), infraspinatus (15%), and subscapularis (5%).[2]
- Calcific tendinosis typically undergoes four stages:[3]
  1. *Precalcific stage*: Initiated by chondral metaplasia of tenocytes within the tendon. This stage may present as dull shoulder pain during the night.
  2. *Calcific stage*: During this stage, there is formation of small calcium deposits. The calcification has "chalk-like" consistency.
  3. *Resorptive stage*: Characterized by increased vascularity and inflammation surrounding the calcific deposit. Phagocytic cells form granulomatous deposits that aid in resorption of the calcium. The calcium typically has

"toothpaste-like" consistency. The patient generally experiences sharp shoulder pain along with restricted shoulder movements.
  4. *Postcalcific stage*: During this stage, fibroblasts migrate to the area of the defect (caused due to calcium resorption) and result in formation of a scar.
- Depending of the stage of calcification, the ultrasound (US) findings may vary. The calcific foci may be seen as:
  - Hyperechoic foci with well-defined acoustic shadowing.
  - Hyperechoic foci with faint shadowing (slurry calcification) (Figs. 1A and B).
  - Hyperechoic foci without shadowing.
- The shape of calcium varies on US. Calcium may be visualized as follows: (1) well-defined chunks, (2) thin hyperechoic strands in the cuff, and (3) semi-liquid calcification (Figs. 2A to C).
- *Role of US in calcific tendinosis*:
  - Localization of calcification within the rotator cuff.
  - Assess the integrity of the cuff.
  - Calculate the distance of calcification from the biceps tendon.
  - *To assess the migration of calcification (Figs. 3A and B)*: Sub-bursal/intrabursal/intraosseous.
  - Ultrasound-guided needling or barbotage of intratendinous calcium is a well-established treatment option for calcific tendinosis.

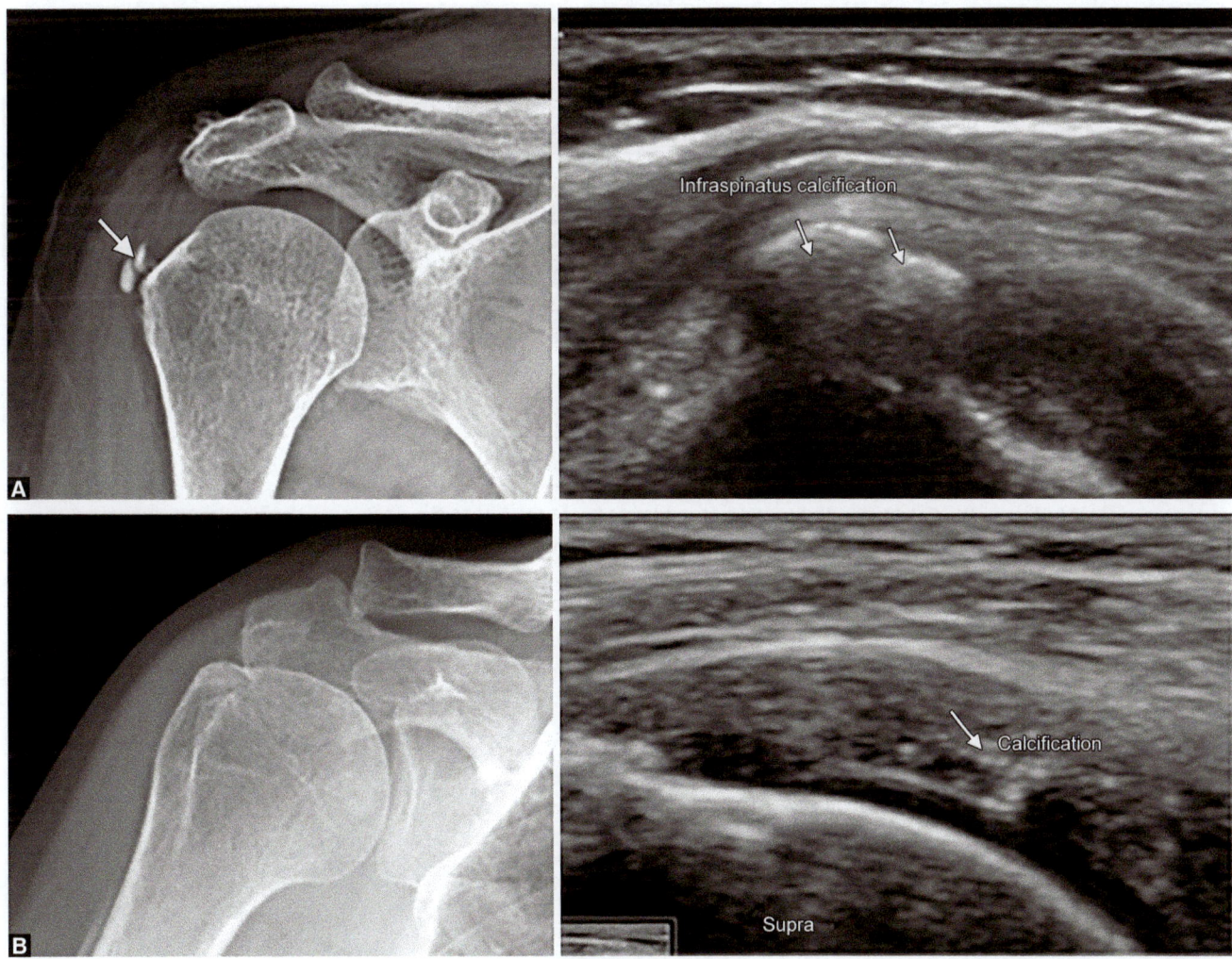

Figs. 2A and B

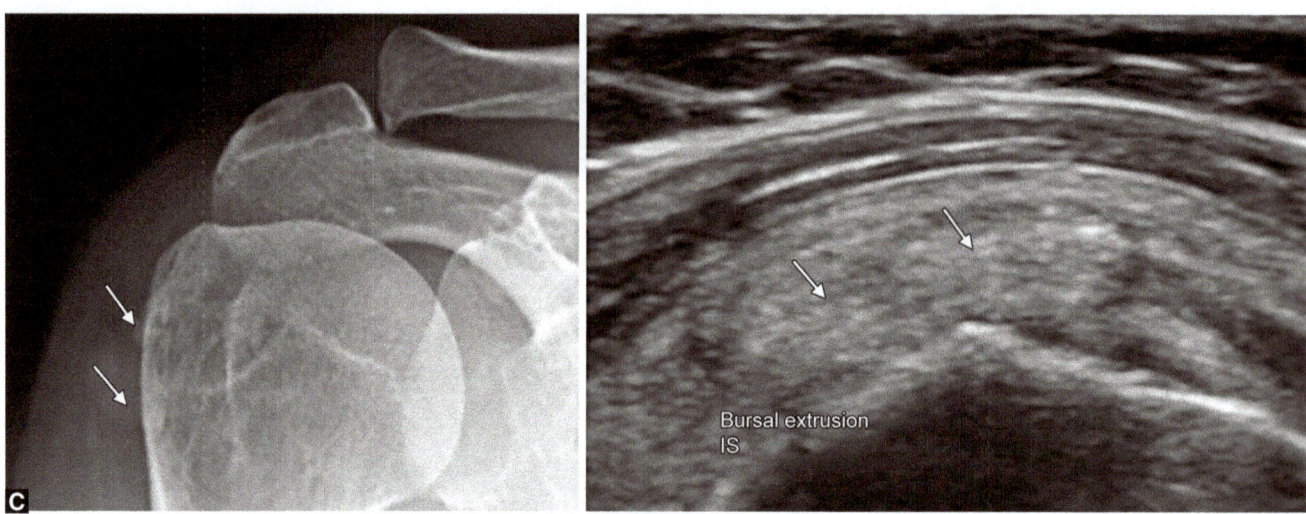

Figs. 2A to C: (A) Well-defined chunks of calcium; (B) Thin hyperechoic strands in the cuff; and (C) Semi-liquid calcification. (IS: infraspinatus)

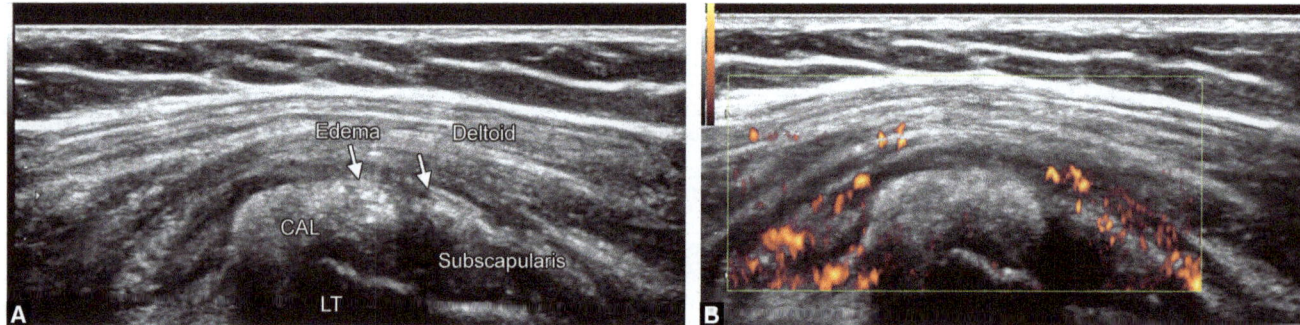

Figs. 3A and B: Extrusion of intratendinous subscapularis calcification (CAL) in the subacromial-subdeltoid bursa results in peribursal edema (arrows) and inflammation. Power Doppler shows and demonstrates neovascularity in the peribursal and intermuscular planes. (LT: lesser tuberosity)

REFERENCES

1. Speed CA, Hazleman BL. Calcific tendinitis of the shoulder. N Engl J Med. 1999;340:1582-4.
2. Mole D, Gonzalvez M, Roche O, et al. Introduction to calcifying tendinitis. In: Gazielly DF, Gleyze P, Thomas T (Eds). The Cuff. France: Elsevier; 1997. pp. 141-3.
3. Bianchi S, Martinoli C. Shoulder. In: Bianchi S, Martinoli C (Eds). Ultrasound of the Musculoskeletal System. Germany: Springer-Verlag; 2007. pp. 190-331.

Case 6

Subacromial-subdeltoid Bursal Inflammation

CLINICAL HISTORY

A 33-year-old lady presented with chronic pain and restricted range of movement in the right shoulder. She is a known case of psoriasis.

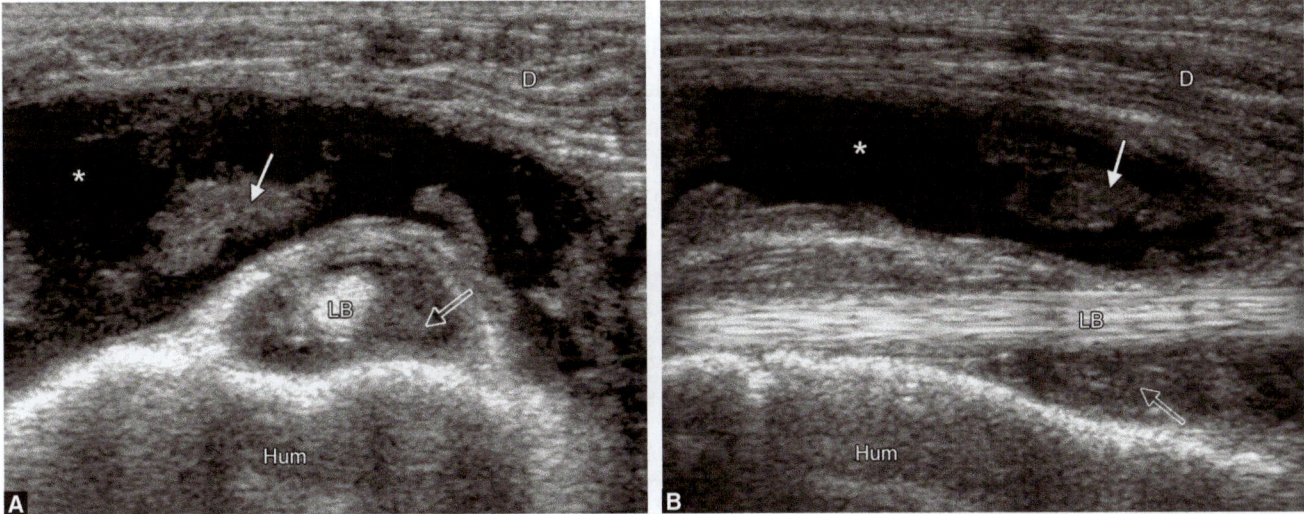

Figs. 1A and B: Transverse and long-axis images of the long head of biceps (LB) show synovial hypertrophy in the biceps tendon sheath (arrow). Moderate volume of anechoic effusion (*) is seen in the subacromial-subdeltoid bursa along with synovial hypertrophy (solid arrow). (Hum: humerus)

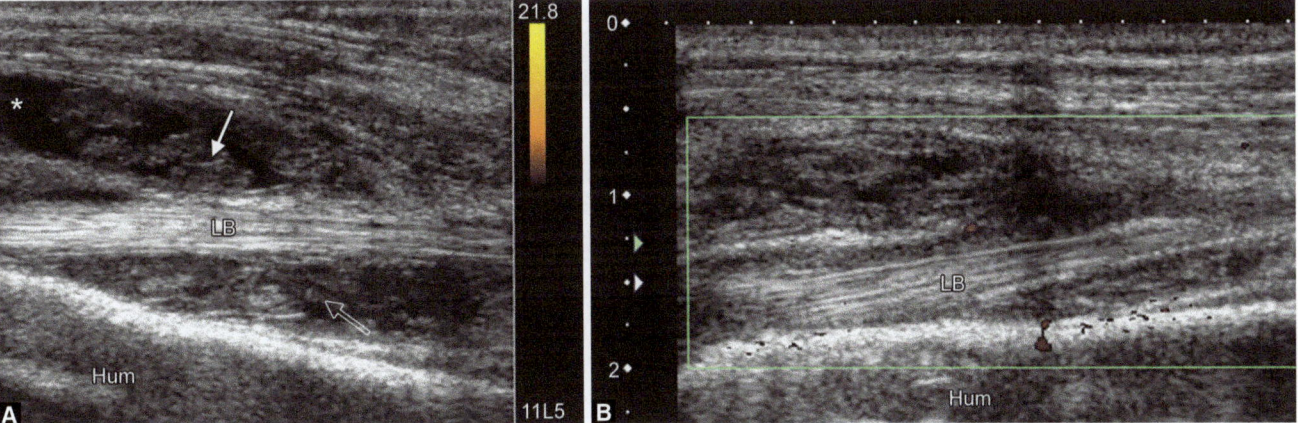

Figs. 2A and B: Long-axis images along with power Doppler of the thickened synovium in the biceps tendon sheath (arrow) and the subacromial-subdeltoid bursa (solid arrow) fail to show any neovascularity. (Hum: humerus; LB: long head of biceps)

DIAGNOSIS

Subacromial-subdeltoid (SASD) bursitis with tenosynovitis of the long head of biceps.

DISCUSSION

- The SASD bursa is a synovium lined cavity that lies above the rotator cuff and below the acromion and deltoid muscle. The bursa allows smooth gliding of the rotator cuff below the coracoacromial arch and the deltoid muscle.
- Laterally, the SASD bursa extends 2 cm beyond the lateral margin of the acromion as it curves around the greater tuberosity. The medial boundary of the SASD bursa lies just below the acromioclavicular (AC) joint. Anteriorly, the SASD bursa lies just over the intertubercular groove.
- Normal SASD bursa measures 2 mm in thickness.[1]
- Inflammation of the SASD bursa is encountered in subacromial impingement syndrome, cuff tears, trauma, inflammatory arthropathies, hydroxyapatite deposition, and infections.[2]
- *Ultrasound (US) findings in SASD bursal inflammation include*:
    - Anechoic or complex bursal fluid resulting in bursal thickness of more than 2 mm.
    - Synovial hypertrophy. Power Doppler may show neovascularity within the thickened synovium (Figs. 1 and 2).
    - Intrabursal loose bodies, i.e. rice bodies, synovial chondromatosis (Figs. 3 and 4), calcium, and lipoma arborescens.
    - Bunching/interrupted sliding of the bursa against the lateral margin of the acromion during shoulder abduction.
    - In refractory cases of shoulder pain, US-guided injection of the SASD bursa has become increasingly popular. Under US guidance, the SASD bursa is injected with a combination of a local anesthetic and a corticosteroid for pain relief and suppression of the inflammation process.

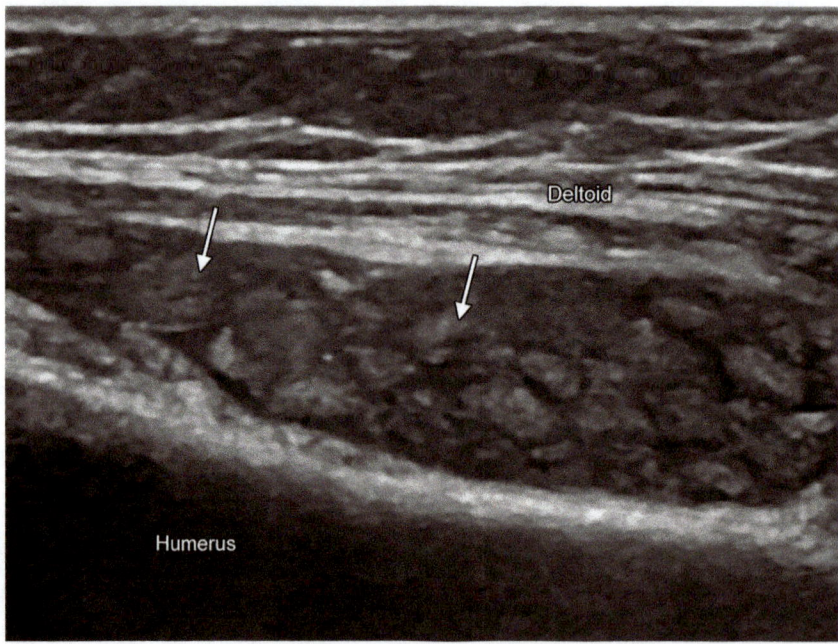

Fig. 3: Long-axis image of the subacromial-subdeltoid bursa shows multiple echogenic nodules (arrows) without any distal shadowing. These findings suggest nodular synovial hypertrophy within the bursa.

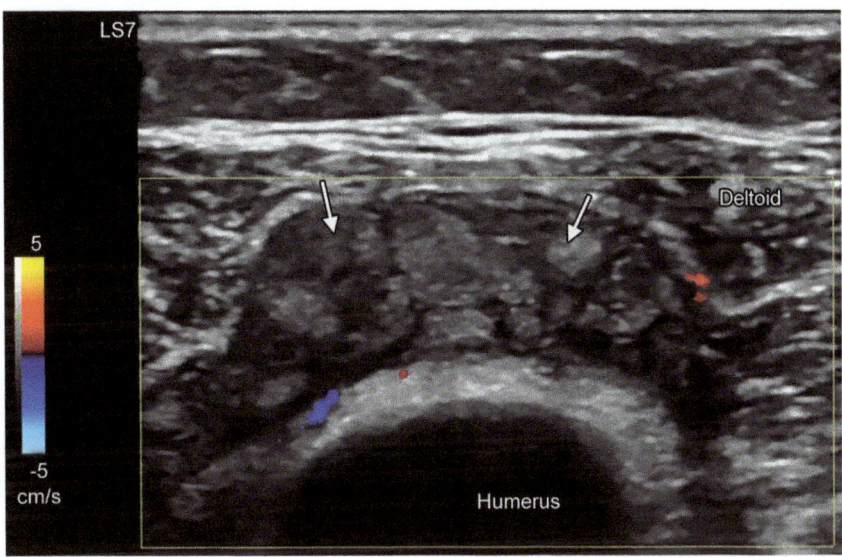

Fig. 4: Transverse image with color Doppler does not show any significant neovascularity within the thickened synovium (arrows).

REFERENCES

1. White E, Schweitzer M, Haims A. Range of normal and abnormal subacromial/subdeltoid bursa fluid. J Comput Assist Tomogr. 2006;30:316-20.
2. Van Holsbeeck M, Strouse PJ. Sonography of the shoulder: evaluation of the subacromial subdeltoid bursa. AJR Am J Roentgenol. 1993;160:561-4.

Case 7

Tear of the Subscapularis Tendon

■ CLINICAL HISTORY

A 62-year-old lady presented with painful internal rotation of the left shoulder. She had sustained a fall on the left hand 8 months ago.

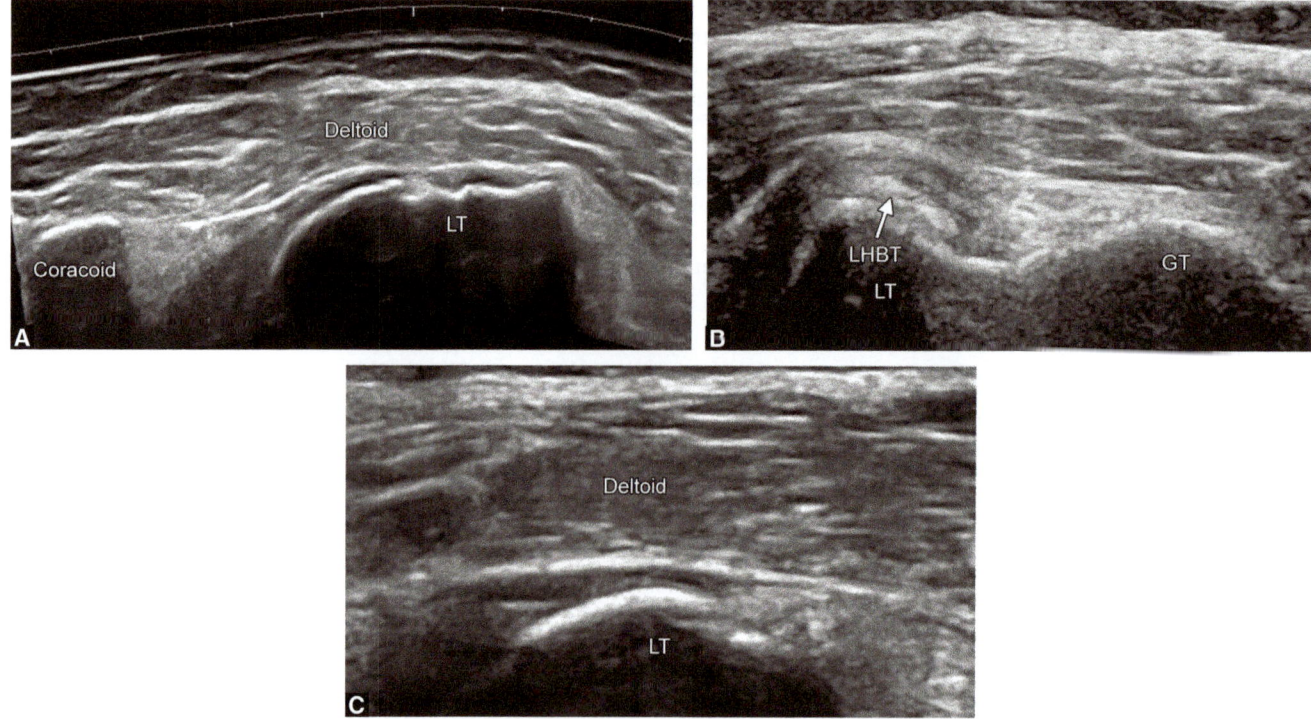

Figs. 1A to C: (A) The subscapularis tendon is not visualized at its expected location between the deltoid and the lesser tuberosity (LT), suggestive of a full-thickness tear with medial retraction of the torn tendon; (B) Full-thickness tear of the subscapularis tendon results in instability of the long head of biceps tendon (LHBT). Transverse image at the level of the bicipital groove shows medial subluxation of the LHBT (arrow); (C) Nonvisualization of the subscapularis tendon between the deltoid and the lesser tuberosity (LT) on transverse images. (GT: greater tuberosity)

Tear of the Subscapularis Tendon

■ DIAGNOSIS

Full-thickness tear of the subscapularis tendon (Figs. 1 and 2).

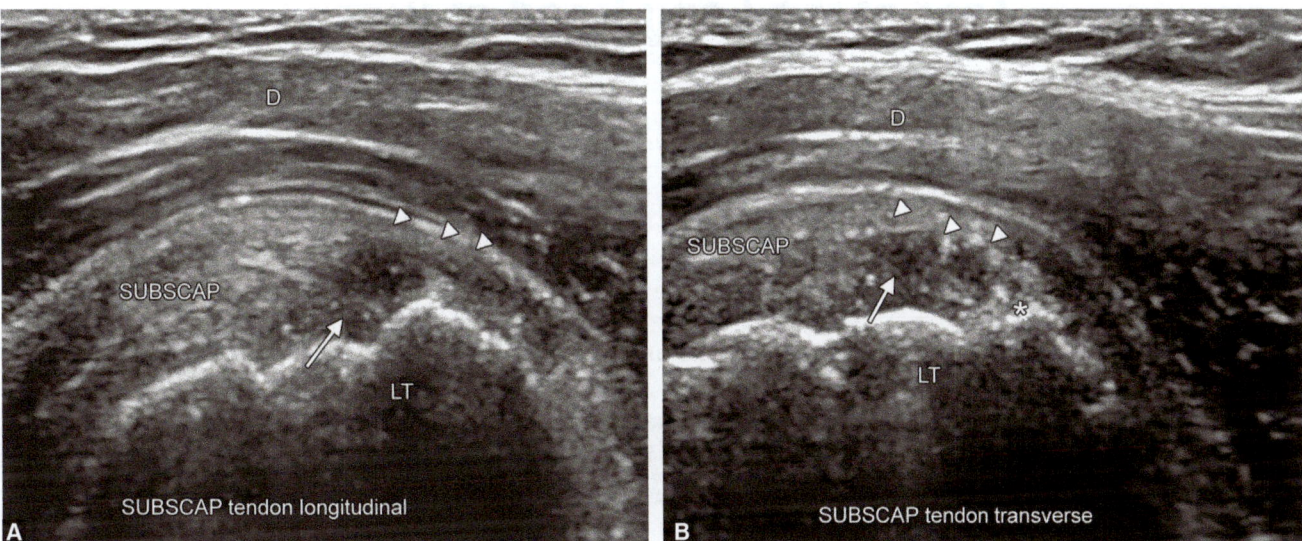

Figs. 2A and B: (A) Long-axis and transverse images show partial-thickness tear (white arrow) involving the deep fibers of the subscapularis (SUBSCAP) tendon; and (B) Cortical irregularity(*) over the lesser tuberosity (LT). Additional case showing a partial thickness tear of the Subscapularis tendon. Arrowheads show intact tendon fibers. (D: deltoid muscle)

Case 8

Tear of the Long Head of Biceps

CLINICAL HISTORY

A 36-year-old man presented with a swelling in the left arm and ipsilateral shoulder since 3 weeks. The injury had occurred while attempting to swing a cricket bat.

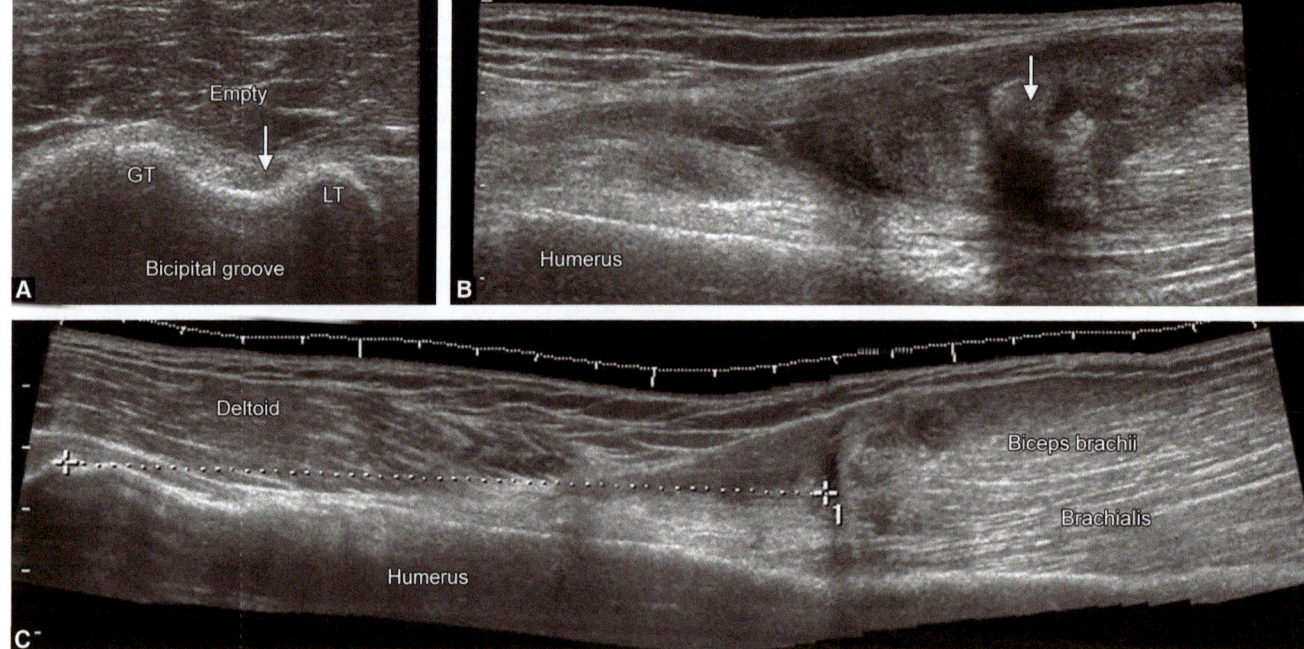

Figs. 1A to C: (A) Transverse image showing an empty bicipital groove (arrow); (B) Extended field of view (EFOV) image along the long-axis of the biceps muscle shows distally retracted biceps tendon. The retracted tendon appears heterogeneous (arrow); and (C) EFOV image is extremely useful for calculation of the distance between the retracted distal biceps tendon and the rotator interval or the proximal tendon stump. (GT: greater tuberosity; LT: lesser tuberosity)

DIAGNOSIS

Rupture of the long head of biceps.

DISCUSSION

- The biceps brachii muscle has two heads. The short head originates from the coracoid process.
- The long head of biceps (LHB) originates from the supraglenoid tubercle. The LHB has an intra-articular as well as an extra-articular course (Fig. 4). The tendon exits the glenohumeral joint through the rotator interval, between the

subscapularis and the supraspinatus tendons. The extra-articular segment of the long head has a tendon sheath, which is an extension of the joint capsule.
- The LHB functions as a dynamic stabilizer of the humeral head.[1]
- The coracohumeral ligament is the primary stabilizer of the LHB at the rotator interval and in the bicipital groove.
- Intrinsic degeneration of the tendon (Figs. 3A and B) or repetitive microtrauma makes the tendon vulnerable to rupture. The tendon commonly tears either at the glenoid insertion or at the level of the proximal intertubercular groove.[2]
- The patient with a full-thickness tear of the LHB commonly presents with a lump along the lateral aspect of the arm following a snapping sensation. This lump is referred to as "Popeye sign".
- Full-thickness tears of the LHB result in loss of elbow supination strength.[3]
- *Ultrasound (US) findings in full-thickness tears of the LHB*:
    - Full-thickness tears of the LHB are seen as discontinuity of the fibers with either a hematoma or fluid.
    - Empty bicipital groove. Nonvisualization of the torn proximal end on US indicates intra-articular retraction of the torn tendon (Figs. 1 and 2).
    - Absence of fibrillar pattern in the bicipital groove.[4] In chronic tears, the echogenic scar tissue in the bicipital groove may be erroneously reported as an intact tendon.
    - Underlying tears of the supraspinatus and subscapularis tendons (Figs. 2A to D).[5]
- **Reporting checklist during US evaluation of full-thickness tear of the LHB:**
    - Size of the tear in static position.
    - Size of the tear with flexion and extension of the elbow.
    - Location of the distal and proximal (if visualized) edges of the tendon.
    - Presence of hematoma.
    - Associated cuff tear.
- The surgical treatment that is generally offered is either tenotomy or tenodesis of the LHB.

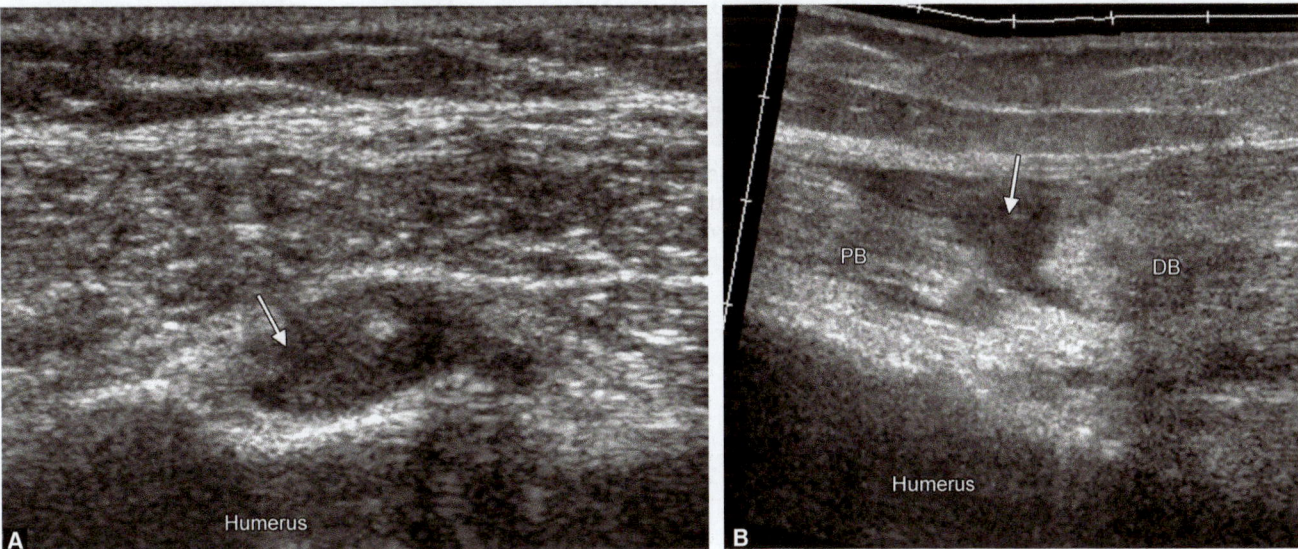

Figs. 2A and B: (A) Transverse image at the level of bicipital groove shows an empty bicipital groove with fluid (arrow); (B) Long-axis image of the biceps tendon shows the proximal (PB) and distal (DB) edges of the torn biceps tendon. The gap (arrow) is filled with fluid.

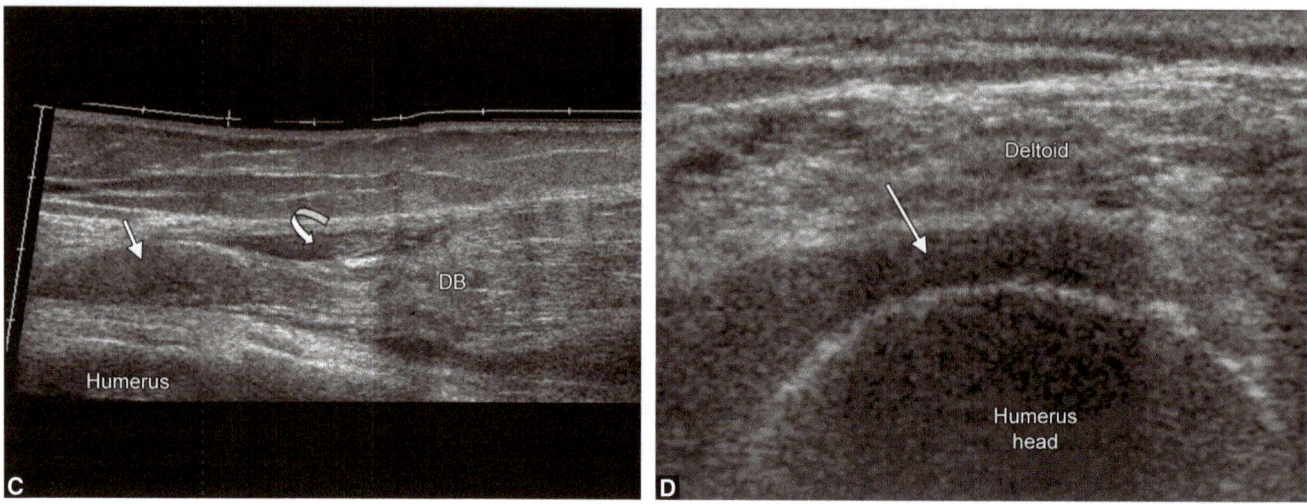

Figs. 2C and D: (C) Extended field of view (EFOV) images along the long-axis of the biceps tendon shows the distal (DB) edge of the torn biceps tendon. The gap (curved arrow) is filled with fluid. The torn DB edge (arrow) appears thickened and hypoechoic—suggestive of underlying tendinosis; (D) Transverse image of the rotator cuff shows nonvisualization of the supraspinatus tendon (arrow) suggestive of an underlying full-thickness tear.

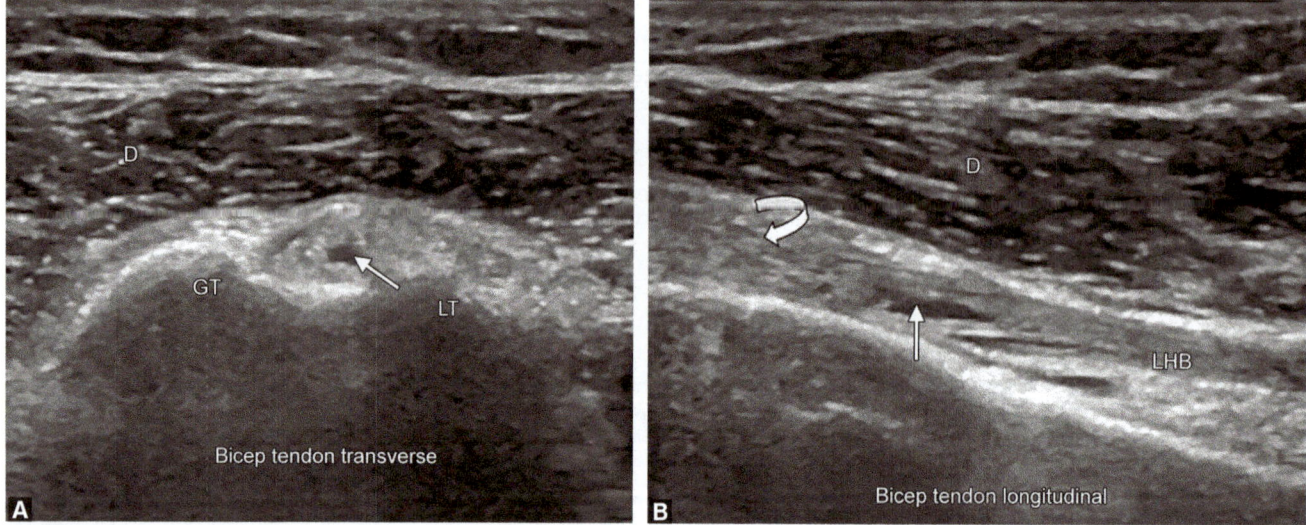

Figs. 3A and B: (A) Transverse and long-axis images at the level of the bicipital groove show a partial-thickness tear (arrow) involving the long head of biceps (LHB); and (B) The proximal fibers of the biceps tendon adjacent to the tear appear hypoechoic (curved arrow). (D: deltoid muscle; GT: greater tuberosity; LT: lesser tuberosity)

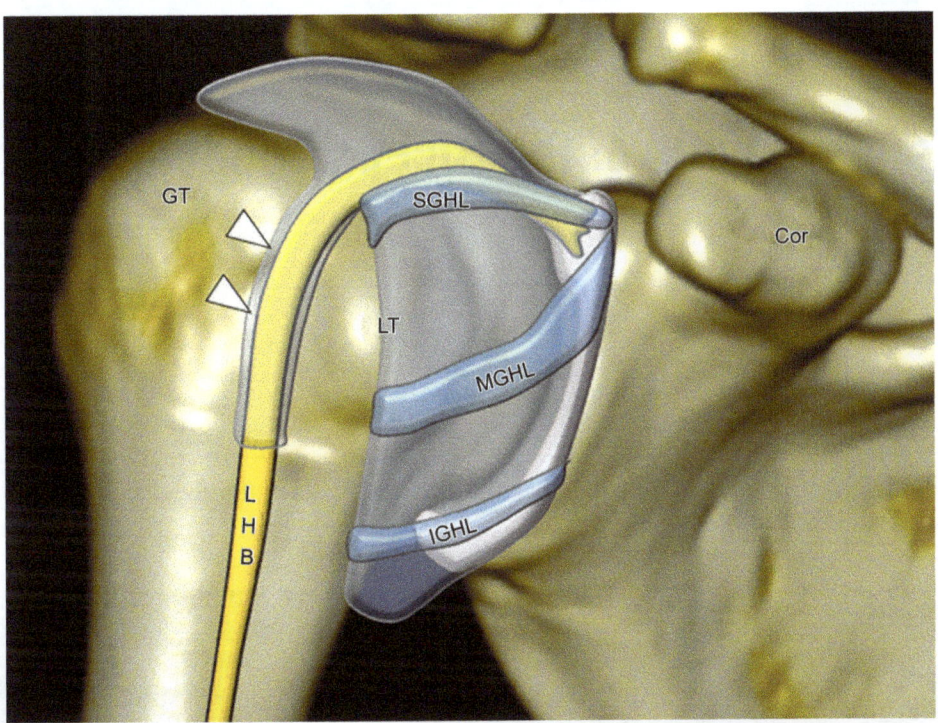

Fig. 4: Course of the long head of biceps (LHB). The LHB is enveloped by the biceps tendon sheath (arrowheads) as it exits the glenohumeral joint through the rotator interval. The glenohumeral ligaments (SGHL, MGHL, and IGHL) are seen as bands of thickened glenohumeral joint capsule. (IGHL: inferior glenohumeral ligament; MGHL: middle glenohumeral ligament; SGHL: superior glenohumeral ligament; Cor: coracoid; LT: lesser tuberosity; GT: greater tuberosity)

REFERENCES

1. Rodosky MW, Harner CD, Fu FH. The role of the long head of the biceps muscle and superior glenoid labrum in anterior stability of the shoulder. Am J Sports Med. 1994;22:121-30.
2. Burkhead WZ, Arcand MA, Zeman C. The biceps tendon. In: Rockwood CA, Matsen FA (Eds). The Shoulder, 3rd edition. Philadelphia: Saunders; 1990.
3. Kelly AM, Drakos MC, Fealy S, et al. Arthroscopic release of the long head of the biceps tendon: functional outcome and clinical results. Am J Sports Med. 2005;33:208-13.
4. Papatheodorou A, Ellinas P, Takis F, et al. US of the shoulder: rotator cuff and non-rotator cuff disorders. Radiographics. 2006;26:e23.
5. Beall DP, Williamson EE, Ly JQ, et al. Association of biceps tendon tears with rotator-cuff abnormalities: degree of correlation with tears of the anterior and superior portions of the rotator cuff. AJR Am J Roentgenol. 2003;180:633-9.

CASE 9

Tenosynovitis of the Biceps Tendon Sheath

■ CLINICAL HISTORY

A 62-year-old woman presented with sharp pain along the anterior aspect of the shoulder since 3 months. She was a known case of rheumatoid arthritis.

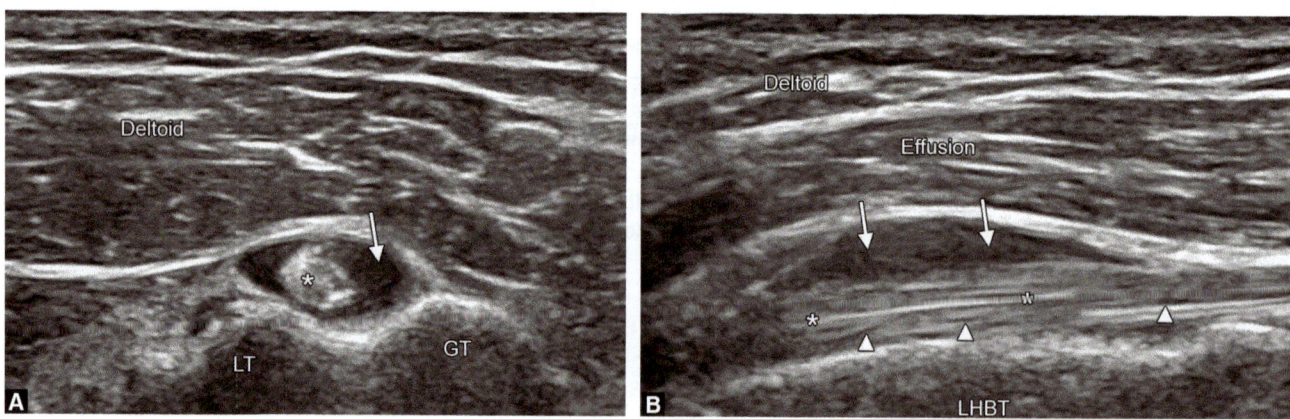

Figs. 1A and B: Transverse and long-axis images at the level of the bicipital groove show anechoic fluid (arrow) surrounding the long head of biceps tendon (LHBT). (LT: lesser tuberosity; GT: greater tuberosity)

■ DIAGNOSIS

Tenosynovitis involving the biceps tendon sheath (Figs. 1A and B).

■ DISCUSSION

- Common causes resulting in tenosynovitis of the biceps tendon sheath are impingement, chronic cuff tears, inflammatory arthritis, and various infections.
- Although ultrasound (US) has a high sensitivity in the diagnosis of biceps tendon sheath effusion, its specificity is quite low.
- *Role of US in biceps tendon sheath tenosynovitis*:
  - Detection of synovial hypertrophy and neovascularity within the tendon sheath which are markers of disease activity.
  - Assessment of integrity of the long head of biceps.
  - Ultrasound guidance for injection of corticosteroid within the biceps tendon sheath.
  - Monitoring disease response.

Case 10

Adhesive Capsulitis of Shoulder

■ CLINICAL HISTORY

A 57-year-old woman presented with a shoulder pain since 4 months. She had restricted range of movements.

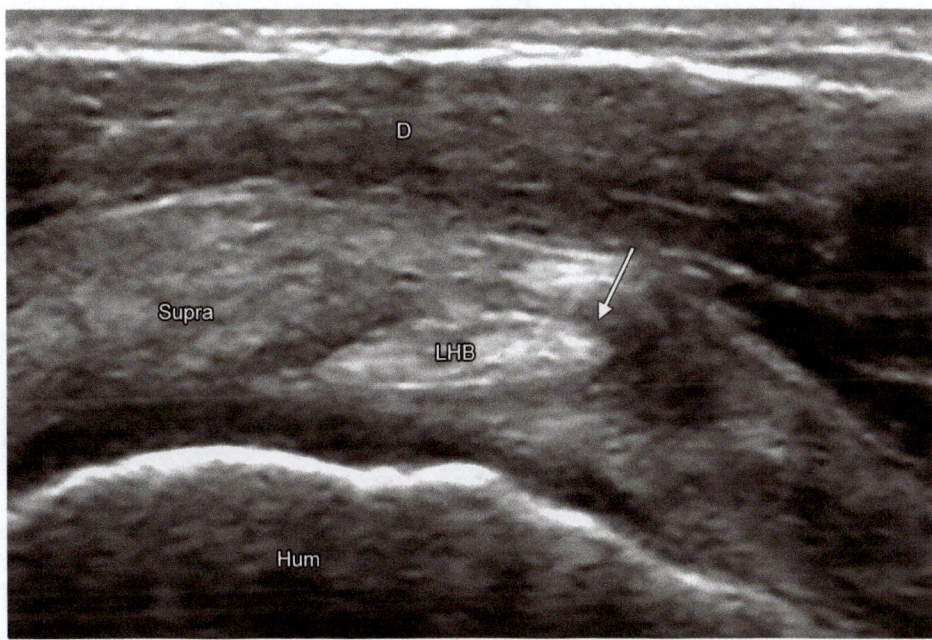

Fig. 1: Transverse image at the level of the rotator interval shows thickened (arrow) coracohumeral ligament.
(D: deltoid muscle; LHB: long head of biceps; Supra: supraspinatus tendon; Hum: humerus)

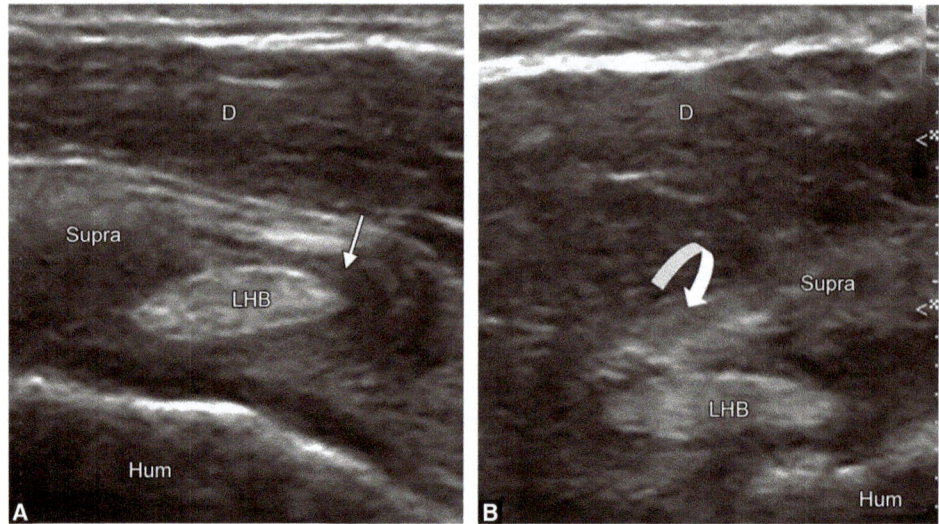

Figs. 2A and B: (A) Transverse image at the level of the rotator interval shows thickened (arrow) coracohumeral ligament; and (B) Comparison with the asymptomatic contralateral shoulder shows echogenic appearance of the normal coracohumeral ligament (curved arrow). (D: deltoid muscle; LHB: long head of biceps; Supra: supraspinatus tendon; Hum: humerus)

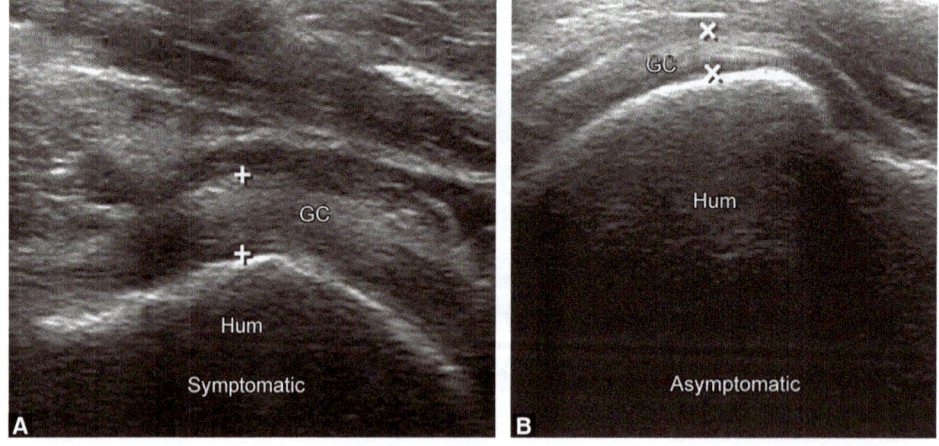

Figs. 3A and B: (A) Figure shows marked thickening of the inferior joint capsule (GC) of the glenohumeral joint; and (B) Comparison with the contralateral side shows normal appearance of the glenohumeral joint capsule. (Hum: humerus; + and ×: position of calipers for measurement of capsule thickness)

DIAGNOSIS

Adhesive capsulitis (AC).

DISCUSSION

- Adhesive capsulitis of shoulder is more commonly referred as "frozen shoulder".

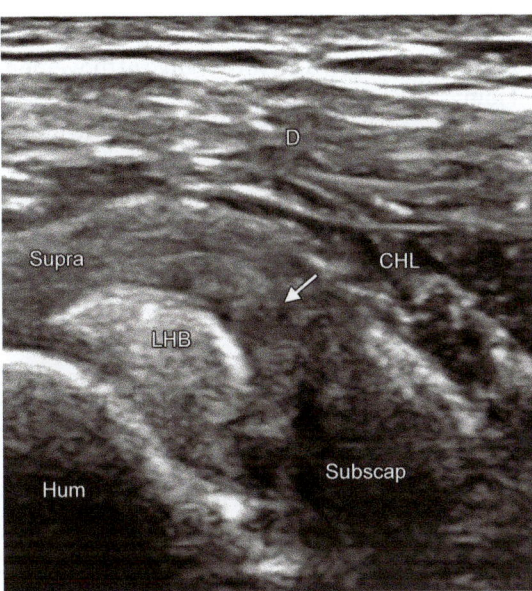

Fig. 4: Transverse image at the level of the rotator interval shows markedly thickened (arrow) coracohumeral ligament (CHL). (D: deltoid muscle; LHB: long head of biceps; Supra: supraspinatus tendon; Hum: Humerus)

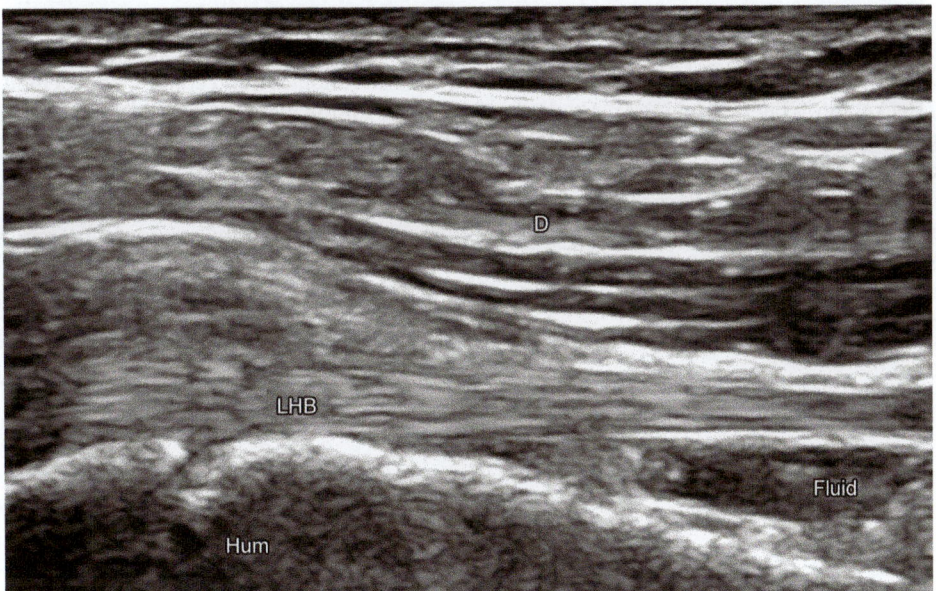

Fig. 5: Long-axis image at the level of the bicipital groove shows anechoic fluid along the long head of biceps tendon (LHB). (D: deltoid muscle; Hum: Humerus)

- Primary AC of the shoulder is characterized by progressive and painful loss of active and passive movements of the shoulder in all directions. Loss of external rotation of the shoulder is a hallmark of this condition.[1] Progressive fibrosis and contracture of the glenohumeral joint capsule is the underlying pathology. It is a self-limiting condition which resolves spontaneously by 2–4 years.[2]
- The incidence of AC is 2–5% in the general population and 10–36% in patients with diabetes mellitus. Women are more commonly affected than men.

- Three stages of primary AC have been described.[3] The stages are as follows:
  1. *Freezing stage*: The patient presents with pain at the end of range of movement. This stage is characterized by acute synovitis of the glenohumeral joint.
  2. *Frozen stage*: Due to the pain at the end of range of motion, there is limited movement of the arm, ultimately resulting in the shoulder being inflexed and internally rotated.
  3. *Thawing stage*: Characterized by improved range of movements.
- Histopathological features of AC include shortening of collagen length, deposition of fibro-fatty tissue in the capsular recesses, collagen bands across joint recesses, production of disorganized collagen, and atrophy of ligaments.[4]
- *Ultrasound (US) findings in AC*:
  - Soft tissue thickening at rotator interval (Fig. 1).
  - Thickening of the coracohumeral ligament more than 3 mm at the rotator interval (Figs. 2 and 4).[5]
  - Increased vascularity in the rotator interval on color Doppler imaging.[6]
  - Mild fluid in the biceps tendon sheath or the subcoracoid recess Fig. 5.
  - Reduced sliding of the supraspinatus tendon below the lateral margin of the acromion on dynamic imaging.
  - Thickened inferior joint capsule (more than 4 mm) (Figs. 3A and B).
  - Secondary AC is due to trauma or sequelae to immobilization.[7]

REFERENCES

1. Calis M, Demir H, Ulker S, et al. Is intraarticular sodium hyaluronate injection an alternative treatment in patients with adhesive capsulitis? Rheumatol Int. 2006;26:536-40.
2. Neviaser AS, Hannafin JA. Adhesive capsulitis: A review of current treatment. Am J Sports Med. 2010;38:2346-56.
3. Hazleman BL. Frozen shoulder. In: Rockwood CA, Matsen FA (Eds). The Shoulder, 2nd edition. Philadelphia: Saunders; 1990.
4. Mangine RE, Heckmann T, Eifert-Mangine M. Alternative techniques for the motion-restricted shoulder. In: Andrews J, Wilk K (Eds). The Athletes Shoulder. New York: Churchill Livingstone; 1994.
5. Homsi C, Bordalo-Rodrigues M, da Silva JJ, et al. Ultrasound in adhesive capsulitis of the shoulder: is assessment of the coracohumeral ligament a valuable diagnostic tool? Skelet Radiol. 2006;35:673-8.
6. Lee JC, Sykes C, Saifuddin A, et al. Adhesive capsulitis: sonographic changes in the rotator cuff interval with arthroscopic correlation. Skelet Radiol. 2005;34:522-7.
7. Malone T, Hazle C. Rehabilitation of adhesive capsulitis. In: Ellenbecker TS (Ed). Shoulder Rehabilitation: Nonoperative Treatment. New York: Thieme; 2006.

Case 11

Paralabral Cyst with Suprascapular Nerve Entrapment

CLINICAL HISTORY

A 32-year-old man presented with a dull aching pain in the left shoulder with difficulty in overhead abduction of the arm.

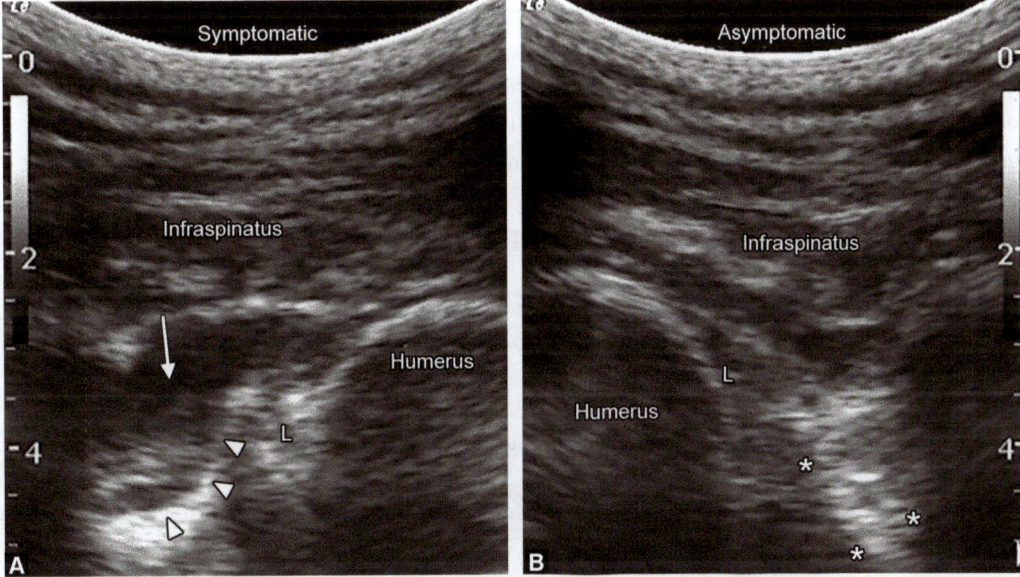

Figs. 1A and B: (A) A long-axis view at the level of the spinoglenoid notch (arrowheads) shows a lobulated cystic lesion (arrow) in close association with the glenoid labrum (L); and (B) The contralateral asymptomatic shoulder and shows normal appearance of the glenoid labrum (L) and the spinoglenoid notch (*).

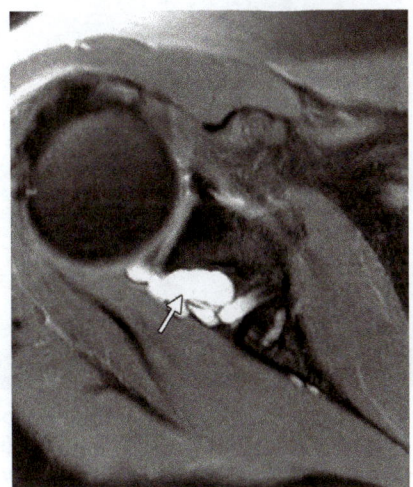

Fig. 2: Axial proton density with fat saturation image of the involved shoulder shows a ganglion (arrow) along the posterior aspect of the labrum extending into the spinoglenoid notch.

DIAGNOSIS

Paralabral cyst resulting in suprascapular nerve entrapment.

DISCUSSION

- The suprascapular nerve (SSN) is a mixed nerve having motor and sensory components. It originates from the upper trunk of the brachial plexus and is formed by C5 and C6 nerve roots. After coursing through the posterior triangle of the neck, it travels the superior margin of the scapula through the suprascapular notch. After innervating the supraspinatus muscle, the nerve enters the infraspinous fossa to innervate the infraspinatus muscle after winding through the spinoglenoid notch (SGN) (Figs. 3A and B).
- Whereas entrapment of the SSN at the level of the suprascapular notch results in denervation of the supraspinatus as well as the infraspinatus muscles, compression of the nerve at the level of the SGN results in isolated denervation of the infraspinatus muscle. Due to difficulty in visualization of the SSN, diagnosis of SSN entrapment is often made by assessing the pattern of muscle atrophy.
- Suprascapular neuropathy is the underlying cause in only 1–2% of the patients with shoulder pain.[1]
- Paralabral ganglion cysts arising from the posterosuperior glenoid labrum are one of the most common causes of SSN entrapment. There is a strong association between a paralabral cyst and a labral tear.[2] Other causes of SSN entrapment include tumors, hematoma, varices, and scapular fractures.[3]
- *Ultrasound (US) findings in paralabral cyst of the shoulder*:
    - Well-defined and lobulated cystic lesion along the posterior aspect of the glenohumeral joint. The unilocular or multilocular cyst may be either anechoic or may contain low-level internal echoes. Power Doppler fails to show any vascularity within the cyst (Figs. 1A and B).
    - The cyst located at the SGN, is closely related to the posterosuperior glenoid labrum (Fig. 2). A hypoechoic cleft representing a labral tear may or may not be visualized.

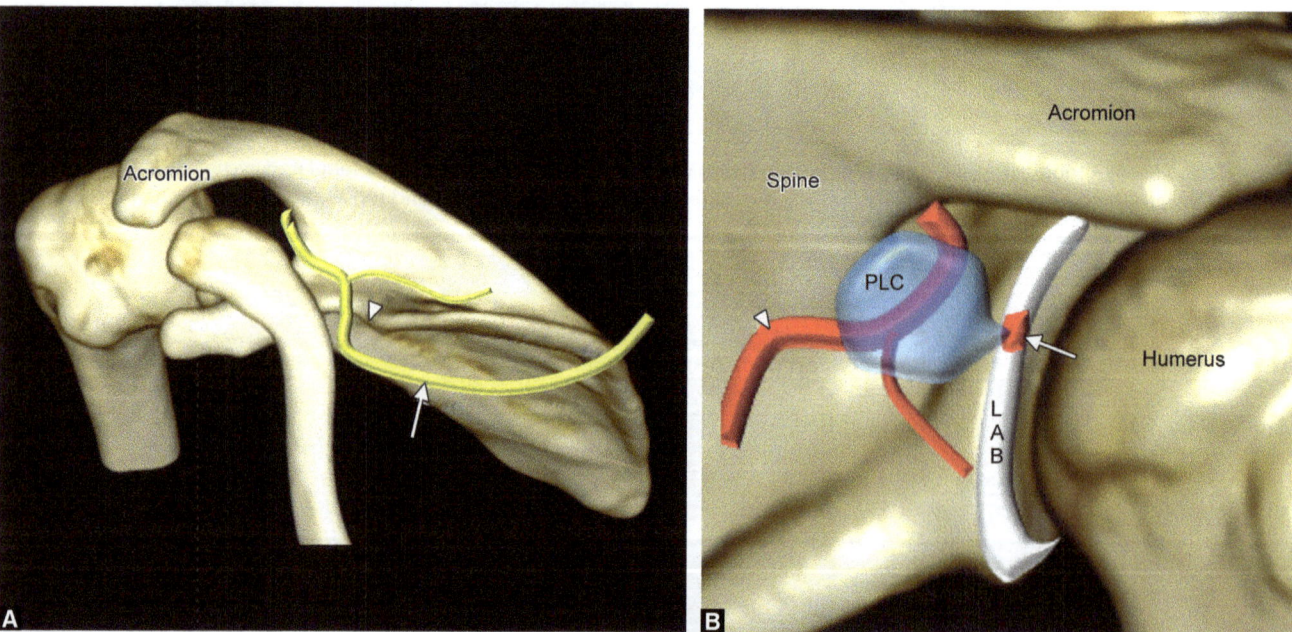

Figs. 3A and B: Paralabral cyst. (A) The course of the suprascapular nerve (arrow) as it courses along the superior margin of the scapula through the suprascapular notch (arrowhead). (B) Paralabral cyst (PLC) arising from a tear (arrowhead) in the posterosuperior labrum (LAB) may compress the nerve (arrow) against the base of the spine at the spinoglenoid notch.

- Atrophy of the infraspinatus muscle may be seen either increased echogenicity (due to fatty atrophy) with preserved muscle volume or increased echogenicity with volume loss. Ipsilateral teres minor muscle or contralateral infraspinatus muscle belly may be used as control.
- Ultrasound-guided aspiration of the paralabral cyst is infrequently done to decompress the nerve.

REFERENCES

1. Boykin RE, Friedman DJ, Higgins LD, et al. Suprascapular neuropathy. J Bone Jt Surg Am. 2010;92:2348-64.
2. Piatt BE, Hawkins RJ, Fritz RC, et al. Clinical evaluation and treatment of spinoglenoid notch ganglion cysts. J Shoulder Elbow Surg. 2002;11:600-4.
3. Fritz RC, Helms CA, Steinbach LS, et al. Suprascapular nerve entrapment: evaluation with MR imaging. Radiology. 1992;182:437-44.

Case 12

Acromioclavicular Joint Dislocation

■ CLINICAL HISTORY

A 23-year-old mixed martial arts player presented a painful swelling over the right shoulder following a fall over the ipsilateral shoulder.

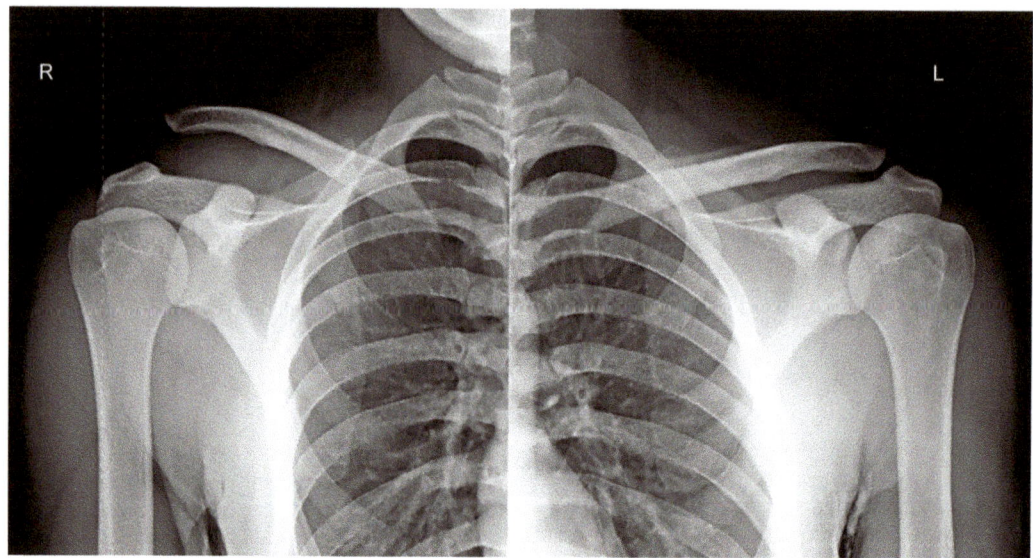

Fig. 1: Frontal stress radiographs of bilateral shoulder joints show dislocation of the right acromioclavicular joint.

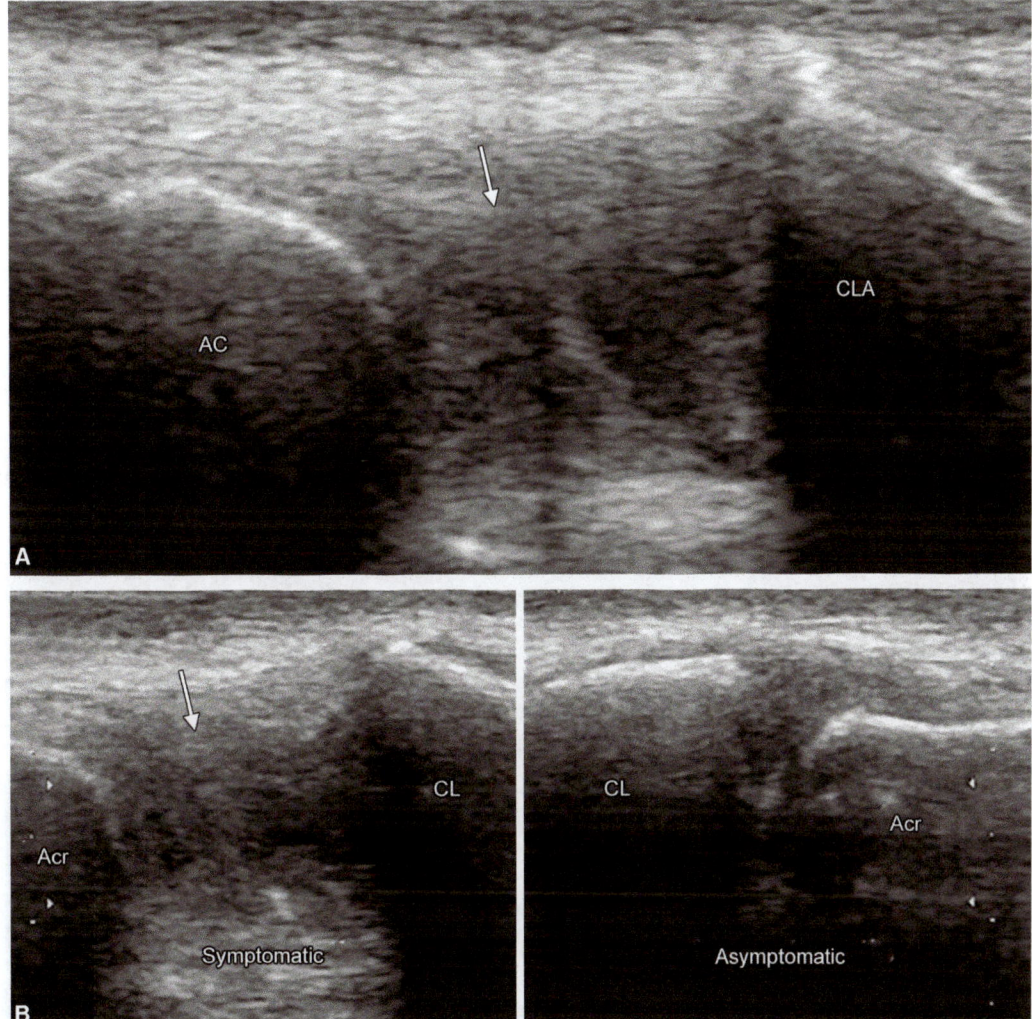

Figs. 2A and B: (A) Transverse image of the right acromioclavicular (AC) joint shows considerable widening of the joint (arrow) along with disruption of the acromioclavicular ligament; and (B) Figure shows comparison with the contralateral (CL) side. (Acr: acromion; CLA: clavicle)

DIAGNOSIS

Acromioclavicular (AC) joint dislocation.

DISCUSSION

- The AC joint is a diarthrodial joint formed by the acromion and the clavicle. A fibrocartilaginous disk is interposed between the two articulating surfaces. The AC joint capsule is relatively weak and is the strongest along its posterosuperior aspect.
- Acromioclavicular joint injuries are most commonly seen in contact sports. The most common classification system used for AC joint injuries is the Rockwood classification.
- *Ultrasound (US) findings in AC joint injuries*:
  - Capsular thickening.
  - Widening of the joint space and altered alignment of the apposing articular surfaces on static and dynamic imaging (Figs. 2A and B).
  - Periarticular edema.
  - Osseous capsular avulsion injuries.
  - Hematoma.
- Unlike magnetic resonance imaging (MRI), the sensitivity and the role of US in the diagnosis of low-grade AC joint injuries is limited. However, it is routinely used for image-guided intra-articular injections for pain management.

Case 13

Traumatic Fat Necrosis

■ CLINICAL HISTORY

A 33-year-old female presented with a painless soft swelling along the superolateral aspect of the right shoulder since 2 months. She has sustained a road traffic accident 1 year ago.

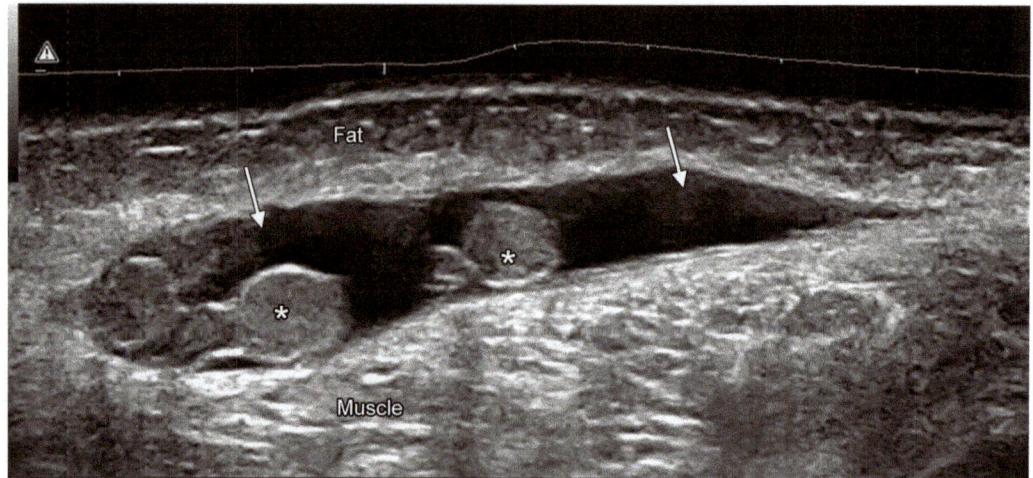

Fig. 1: Long-axis image shows a well-localized complex (arrows) collection between the subcutaneous fat and the muscle. Well-defined echogenic nodules (*) are seen within the collection.

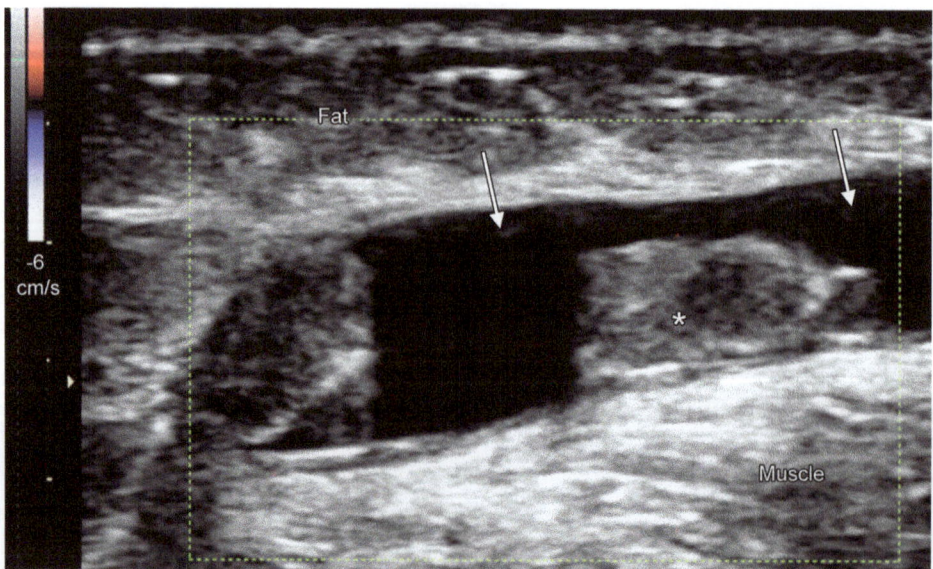

Fig. 2: Power Doppler does not show any vascularity within echogenic nodules. Fat lobules (*).

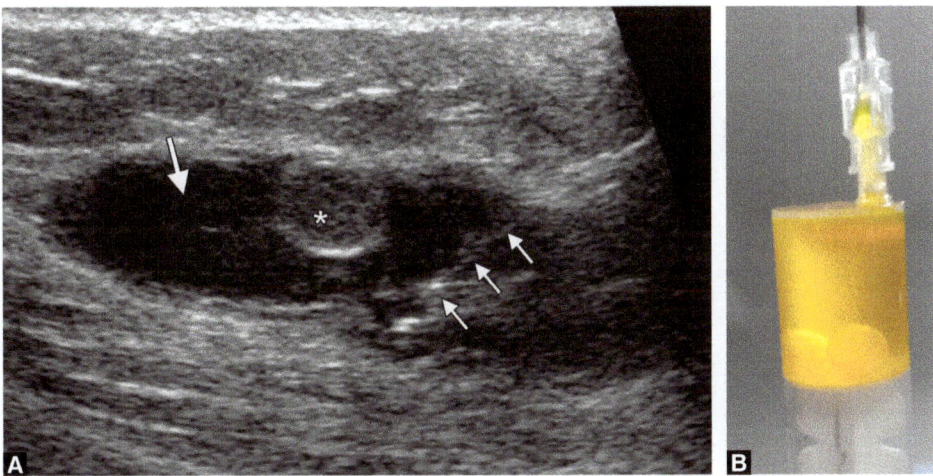

Figs. 3A and B: Ultrasound-guided aspiration of the collection yielded oily fluid with globules (*); (Figure B), suggestive of liquefied fat.

DIAGNOSIS

Traumatic fat necrosis (TFN).

DISCUSSION

- Appendicular TFN may mimic soft tissue tumors. Traumatic foot necrosis (TFN) is often seen over osseous prominences.
- History of obvious trauma may or may not be recalled by the patient.
- In the post-traumatic event, the lipase released by the blood and soft tissue results in aseptic saponification of the fat.
- Ultrasound (US) appearance of TFN is quite variable.[1]
- *US features of TFN include:*
  - Hypoechoic areas within the fat surrounded by an echogenic rim.
  - Isoechoic area bounded by a hypoechoic rim.
  - Edema between the hyperechoic or hypoechoic fat lobules.
  - Encapsulated hypoechoic collection between the echogenic fat lobules. This finding is more commonly seen in the setting of an internal degloving injury (Figs. 1 to 3).[2]

REFERENCES

1. Robinson P, Farrant JM, Bourke G, et al. Ultrasound and MRI findings in appendicular and truncal fat necrosis. Skeletal Radiol. 2008;37:217-24.
2. Parra JA, Fernandez MA, Encinas B, et al. Morel-Lavallée effusions in the thigh. Skeletal Radiol. 1997;26:239-41.

CASE 14

Radial and Ulnar Nerve Injury

CLINICAL HISTORY

A 58-year-old female presented inability to move her fingers following a crush injury over the arm (Fig. 1).

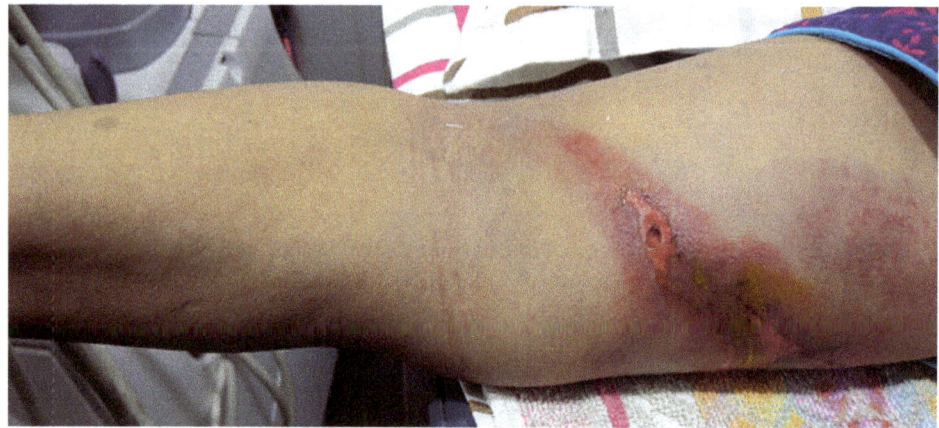

Fig. 1: A puncture wound is seen along the anteromedial aspect of the distal arm.

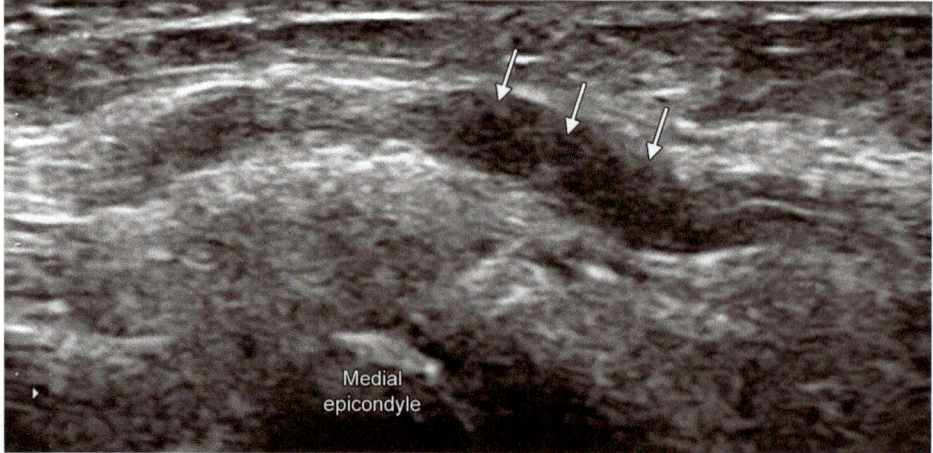

Fig. 2: Long-axis image at the level of the distal arm shows a short segment (arrows) of the ulnar nerve to be thickened and hypoechoic without any discontinuity of the fibers.

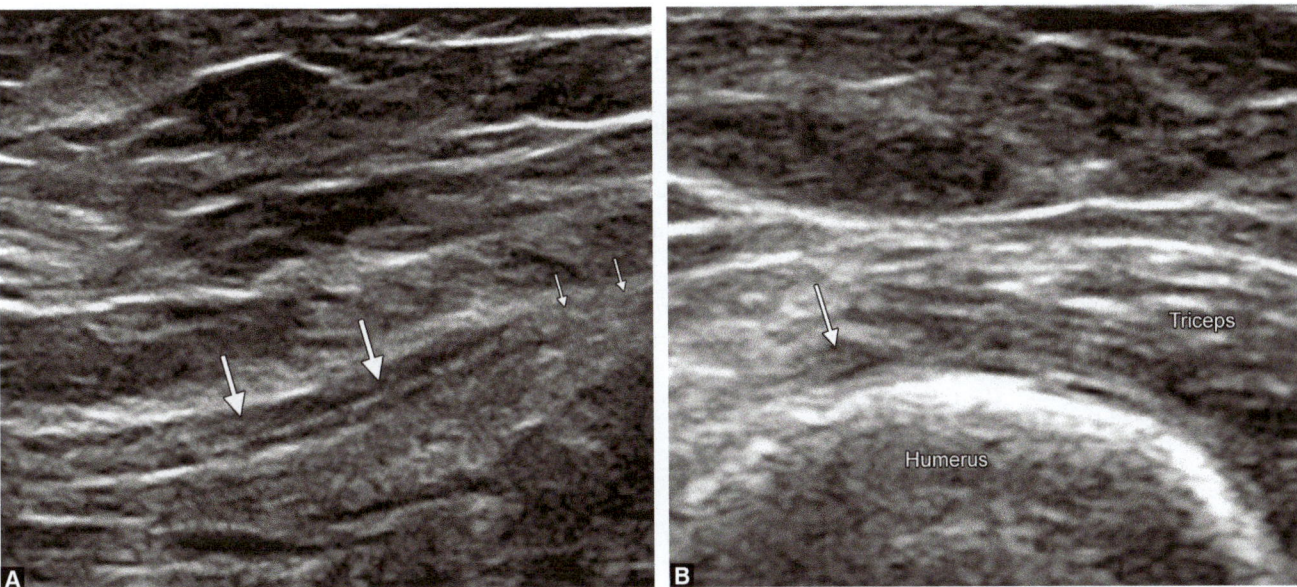

Figs. 3A and B: (A) Long-axis image of the radial nerve shows segmental thickening (thick arrows) of the radial nerve. The nerve proximal to this segment appears normal (thin arrows); and (B) Axial image shows mild thickening of the radial nerve (arrow) at the level of the spiral groove.

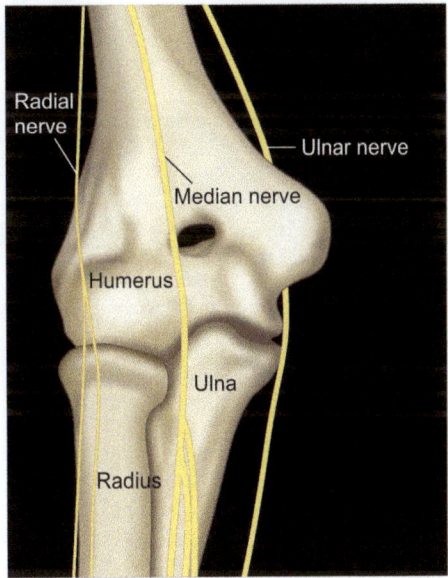

Fig. 4: Nerves traversing the elbow.

DIAGNOSIS

Contusion of ulnar and radial nerves.

DISCUSSION

- Traumatic nerve injuries are broadly categorized as stretching injuries, nerve contusions, and penetrating wounds.
- Stretching nerve injuries occur due to recurrent traction and overuse activities. Ultrasound (US) imaging findings of stretching nerve injuries include discontinuity of the fascicles with a preserved nerve sheath. The nerve may have a wavy contour (Fig. 2).

- On delayed US scans, involved segment of the nerve may show fusiform enlargement due to development of a neuroma.
- Contusion injuries occur where a nerve is closely related to an osseous prominence. Fusiform thickening of the involved segment of the nerve is seen on US (Figs. 3A and B).
- Penetrating injuries may cause partial or complete discontinuity of the nerve fascicles. In long-standing cases, a neuroma typically develops at the site of nerve injury.
- *Role of US in evaluation of traumatic injuries to nerve*:
  - Detection and characterization of abnormal nerve morphology.
  - Assessment of integrity of the nerve sheath.
  - Assessment of the distance between the torn ends of the nerve in presence of a complete tear.

Case 15

Stretch Injury of the Radial Nerve

CLINICAL HISTORY

A 72-year-old female presented with wrist drop in the immediate postoperative period following internal fixation of a fracture of the humeral shaft (Fig. 1). The surgery was performed 1 month ago.

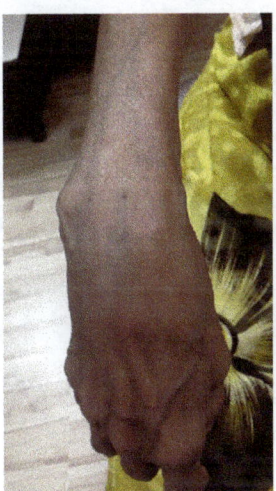

Fig. 1: Clinical photograph shows wrist drop.

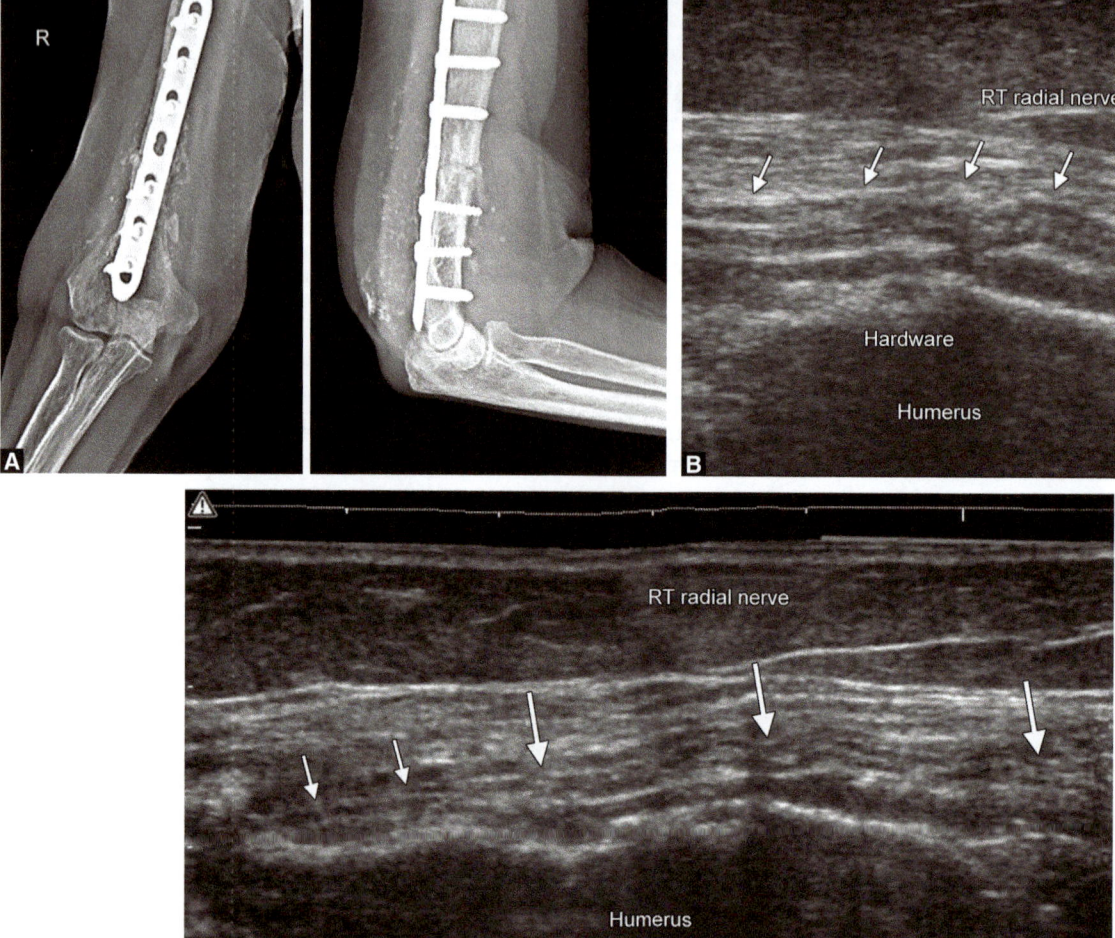

Figs. 2A to C: (A) Frontal and lateral radiographs show the position of metallic implants and morphology of the fracture; (B) Long-axis image shows mild thickening and waviness of the radial nerve (arrows) as it traverses the fracture site; and (C) Long-axis extended field of view shows mild thickening of the radial nerve (thick arrows) as it traverses the fracture site. The distal segment of the nerve (small arrows) is normal in caliber. There is no discontinuity of the nerve fibers. (RT: right)

■ DIAGNOSIS

Stretch injury of the radial nerve due to repeated handling of the nerve during surgery.

Case 16

Intramuscular Cysticercosis of the Triceps Muscle Belly

CLINICAL HISTORY

An 18-year-old female presented with a painless palpable lump along the posterior aspect of the arm.

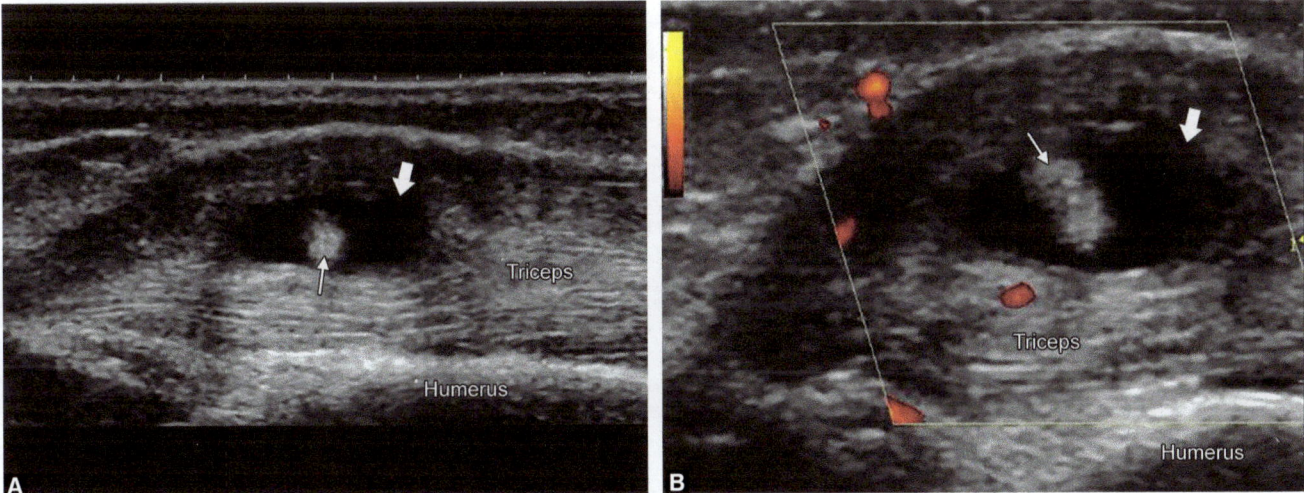

Figs. 1A and B: A well-defined cystic lesion (thick arrow) is seen in the triceps muscle belly along with a central echogenic nodule (thin arrow). The nodule represents the scolex within the cysticercus. Power Doppler image shows mild vascularity in the perilesional muscle fibers.

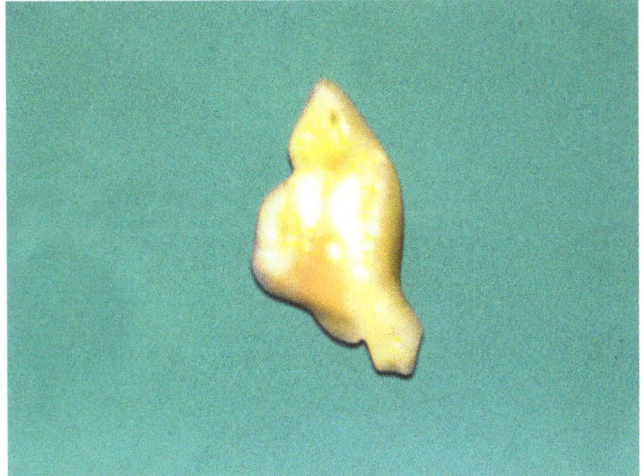

Fig. 2: Gross appearance of the excised cysticercus.

DIAGNOSIS

Intramuscular cysticercosis involving the triceps muscle belly.

DISCUSSION

- Cysticercosis is an infection caused by encysted larvae of *Taenia solium*.
- Cysticercosis may involve any part of the body, particularly the brain, spinal cord, orbit, skeletal muscles, and the myocardium.
- On ultrasound (US) examination, the cysticercus is typically seen as a well-defined cyst with a central echogenic nodule. The central echogenic nodule represents the scolex (Figs. 1A and B).
- In case of partial rupture of the cysticercus, anechoic fluid is seen surrounding the cysticercus. Secondary inflammation or infection of the cysticercus may result in abscess formation.
- Rarely, only a cyst may be seen on US without any evidence of a central scolex. This appearance is thought to be either due to extrusion of the scolex or partial collapse of the cyst due to death of the larva.

CASE 17

Ulnar Nerve Neuritis

CLINICAL HISTORY

A 24-year-old man presented with sensory neuropathy of the right upper limb along the distribution of the ulnar nerve.

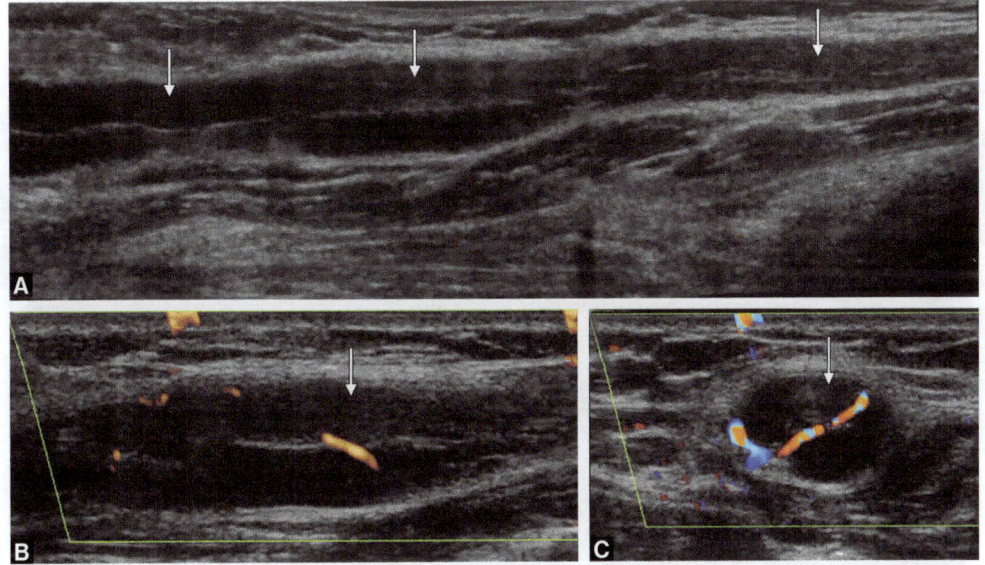

Figs. 1A to C: Long-axis and transverse images show diffuse thickening of the ulnar nerve (arrows). The nerve appears diffusely hypoechoic. Color Doppler images show marked intraneural vascularity.

DIAGNOSIS

Ulnar neuritis (due to leprosy).

DISCUSSION

- Leprosy, also known as Hansen disease, is a chronic granulomatous infection caused by *Mycobacterium leprae*.
- The infection typically involves the skin and the nerves.
- There are three broad forms of leprosy—(1) tuberculoid type, (2) lepromatous type, and (3) intermediate type. Tuberculoid variant of the infection is characterized by aggressive inflammation of the nerve, wherein there is thickening of epineurium and perineurium along with destruction of nerve fascicles. In the lepromatous variant of infection, the inflammation is slow and more prolonged with preservation of the nerve.
- Ulnar nerve, median nerve, and the common peroneal nerve are the commonly affected nerves.
- *Ultrasound (US) findings*:
  - Nerve thickening and hypoechogenicity of the perineurium.
  - Loss of the fascicular pattern (Figs. 1A to C).
  - Intraneural hyperemia on color and power Doppler imaging.
  - Abscess originating from the nerve.

Case 18

Olecranon Bursitis

■ CLINICAL HISTORY

A 50-year-old male presented with a slowly increasing swelling over the posterior aspect of the elbow since 6 years.

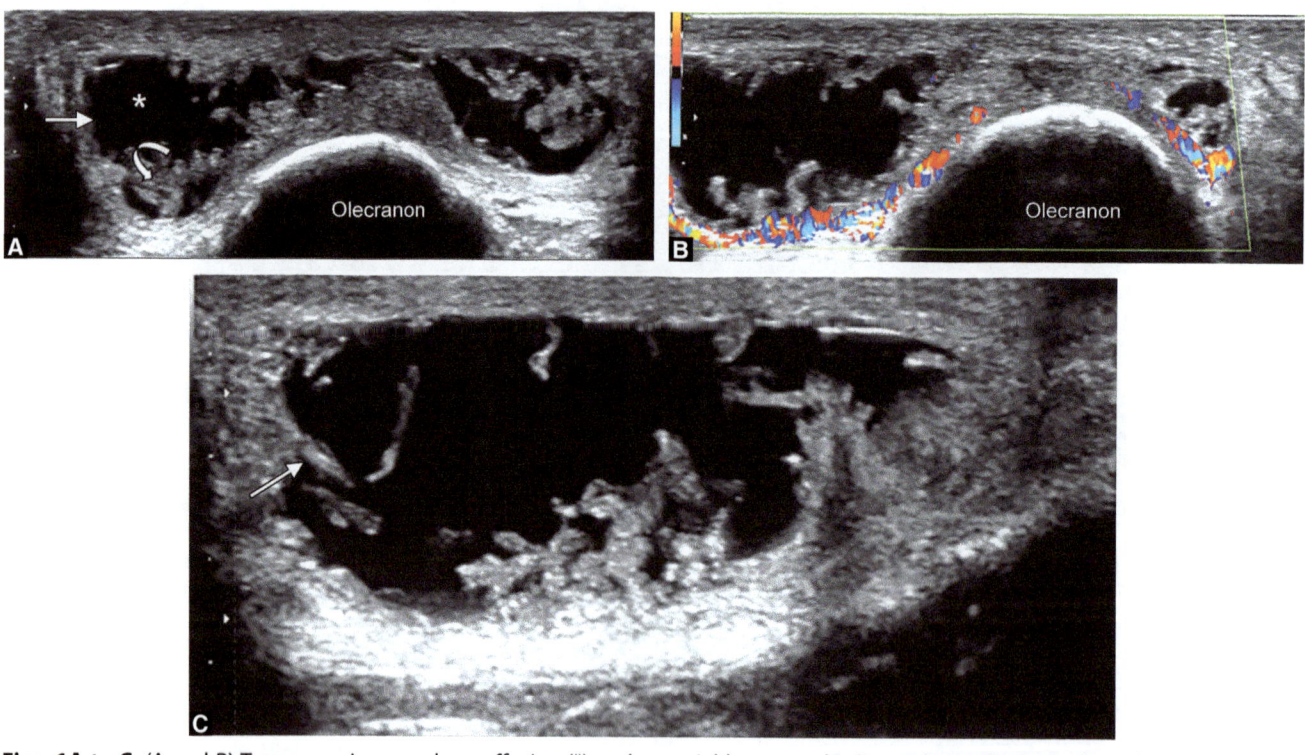

Figs. 1A to C: (A and B) Transverse images show effusion (*) and synovial hypertrophy (curved arrow) within the enlarged olecranon bursa (arrow). Color Doppler shows marked vascularity at the periphery of the thickened synovium; and (C) The enlarged olecranon bursa (arrow) on the long axis.

DIAGNOSIS

Olecranon bursitis.

DISCUSSION

- The olecranon bursa is an anatomical bursa that lies between the olecranon process of the ulna and the subcutaneous fat. It is the most commonly affected bursa in the elbow joint.
- Chronic microtrauma is the most common cause of olecranon bursitis. Crystal deposition disease and inflammatory arthropathies are the other common causes resulting in bursal inflammation.
- On ultrasound (US), the inflamed olecranon bursa may either be seen as a cystic structure (with or without synovial hypertrophy) or as a thickened hypoechoic soft tissue lying in close approximation with the olecranon process (Figs. 1A to C).
- Power Doppler shows increased flow within the hypertrophied synovium when the bursa is inflamed (Figs. 2A to C).
- Occasionally, a loose body may also be seen in the thickened olecranon bursa.

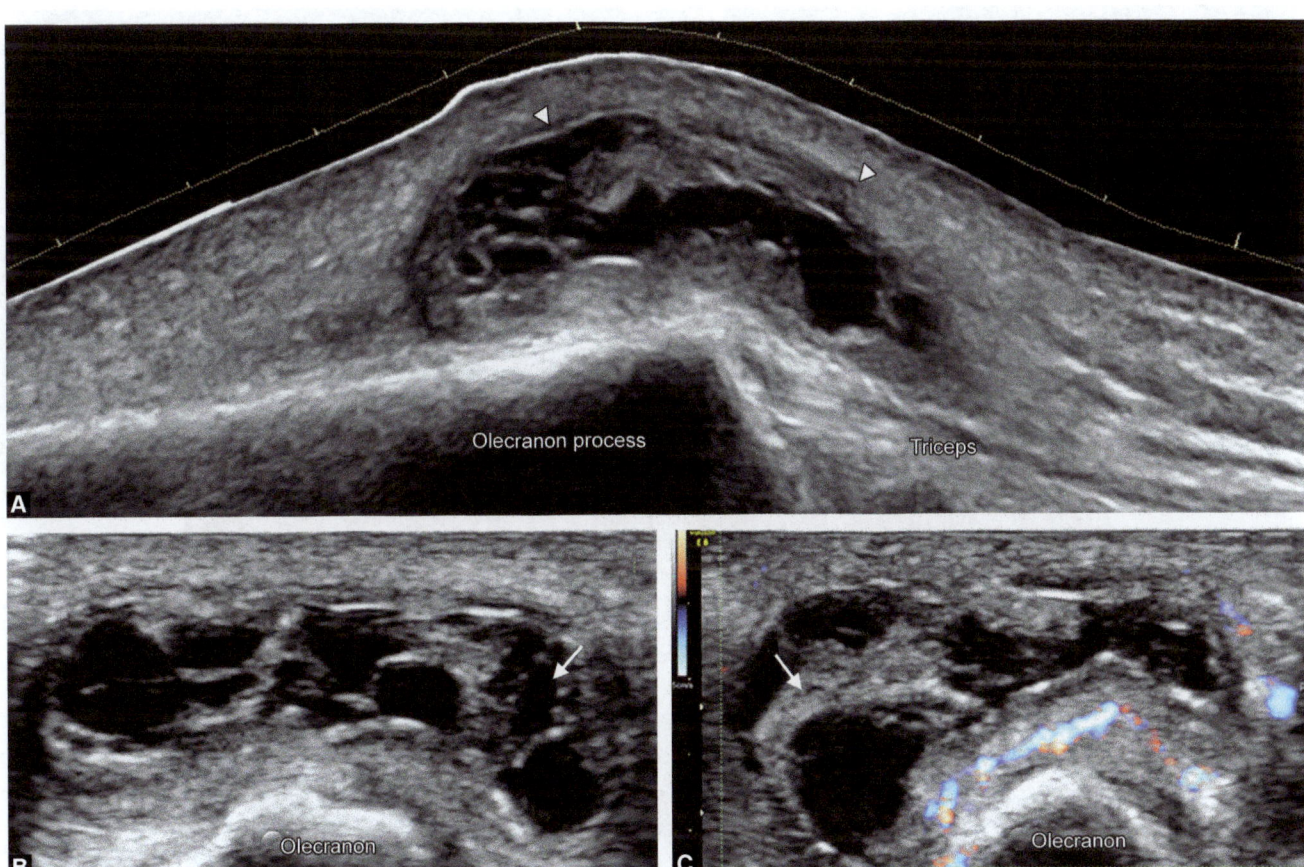

Figs. 2A to C: (A) Extended field of view along the long axis shows the inflamed olecranon bursa (arrowheads) located between the subcutaneous fat above and the olecranon process and the triceps tendon below; and (B and C) Transverse images show the bursa (arrow) to have multiple septae, hypertrophied synovium, and complex fluid. Power Doppler shows neovascularity along the bursal walls.

Case 19

Bicipitoradial Bursitis

CLINICAL HISTORY

A 51-year-old female presented with pain along the anterior aspect of the elbow since 1 month. She was diagnosed to have chikungunya viral infection 2 years ago.

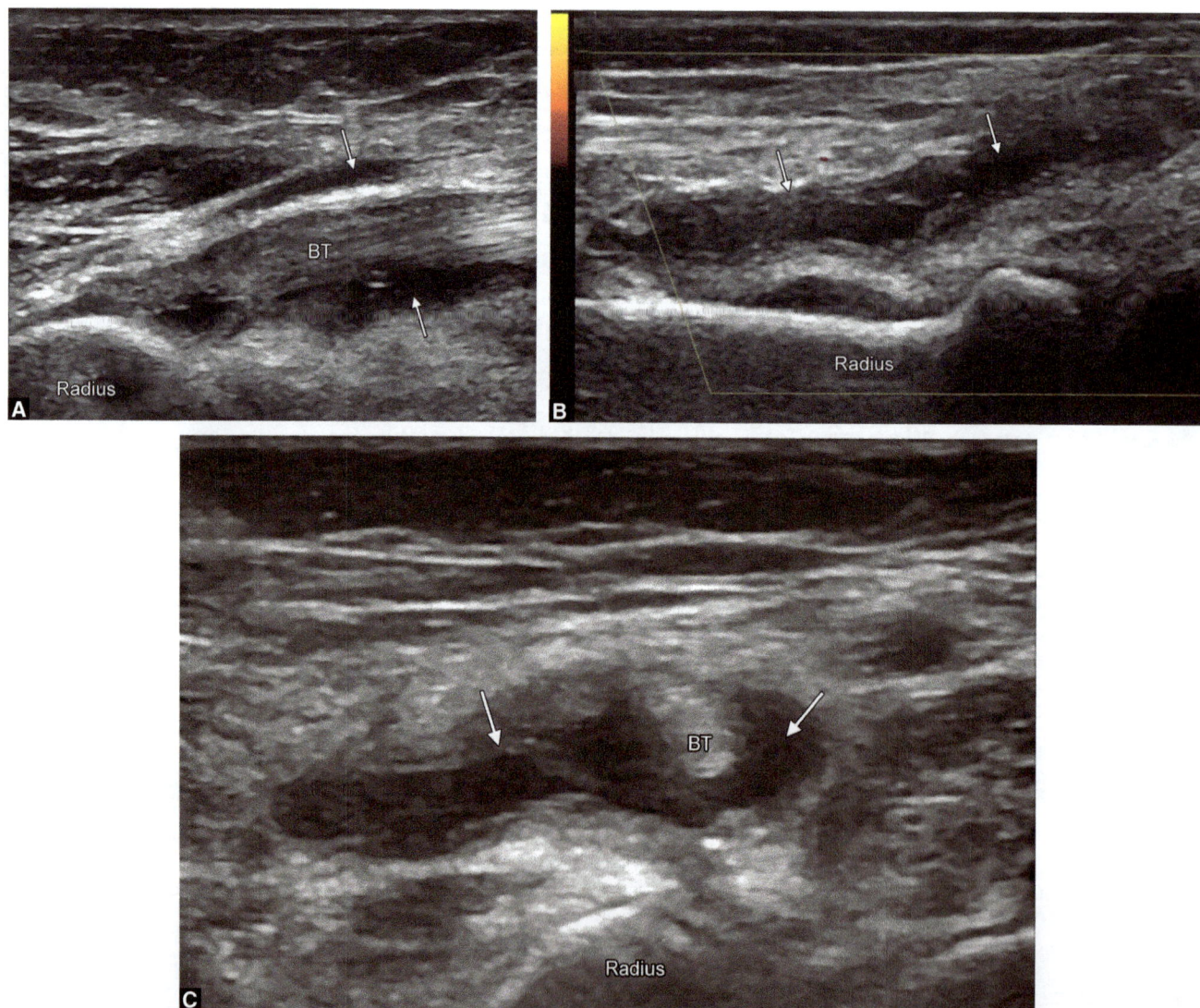

Figs. 1A to C: (A and B) Long-axis images show fluid (arrows) surrounding the distal biceps tendon (BT). Heterogeneous echotexture of the peri-insertional fibers of the distal BT is due to anisotropy. Figure B shows mild synovial hypertrophy within the bicipitoradial bursa without any significant neovascularity on power Doppler; and (C) Transverse image shows the bicipitoradial bursa (arrows) encircling the distal BT.

DIAGNOSIS

Bicipitoradial bursitis (BRB).

DISCUSSION

- The BRB is located along the anterior aspect of the proximal forearm between the distal biceps tendon and the radial tuberosity. The bursa encases the distal biceps tendon (Figs. 1A to C) during supination and gets compressed between the biceps tendon and the radial tuberosity during pronation.
- Just like the bursae elsewhere in the body, the BRB may be affected by either mechanical, inflammatory, or infective etiology. Bursal enlargement is also seen when there is synovial metaplasia or in presence of a pseudotumor (e.g. pigmented villonodular synovitis, lipoma).

Case 20

Tennis Elbow

■ CLINICAL HISTORY

A 41-year-old laborer with 6 weeks history of left elbow pain. The pain was aggravated on lifting a heavy object.

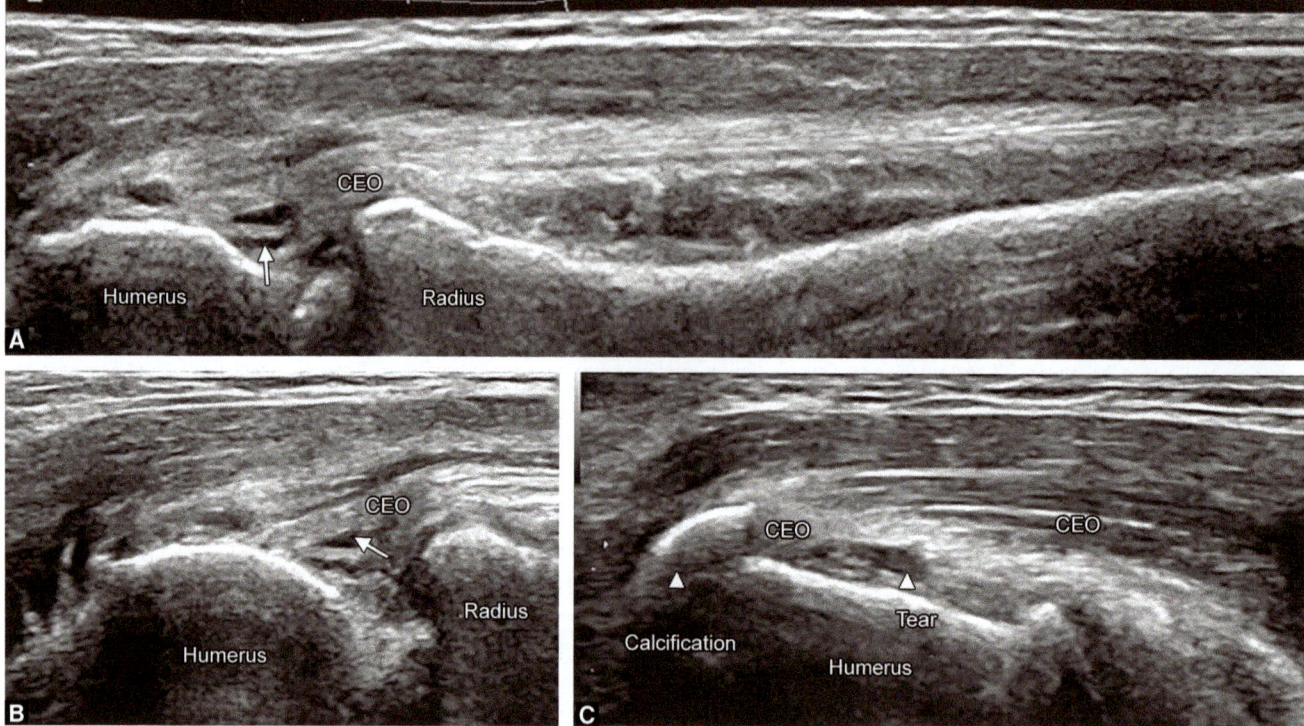

Figs. 1A to C: Long-axis and transverse images show partial-thickness tears (arrow) in the deep fibers of the common extensor origin (CEO). Transverse view also shows focal calcification (arrowheads) in the peri-insertional fibers of the common extensor origin tendon.

■ DIAGNOSIS

Partial-thickness tears involving deep fibers of the common extensor origin (tennis elbow).

■ DISCUSSION

- Tennis elbow or lateral epicondylitis is characterized by pain along the lateral aspect of the elbow and is considered as an overuse injury to the tendons of the common extensor tendon (CET). This condition is prevalent in athletes as well as the nonsporting population.

- Extensor carpi radialis brevis (ECRB), extensor digitorum communis (EDC), and the extensor carpi ulnaris (ECU) form a conjoined tendon as they arise from the lateral epicondyle of the humerus. The CET is formed by the conjoined tendon and the extensor digiti minimi.[1]
- At the lateral epicondyle, CET is arranged in two layers. EDC forms the superficial layer of the CET. The deeper layer is formed by the ECRB. The ECRB lies just above the lateral collateral ligament (LCL) and is intimately related to it with the help of crossing fibers.[1]
- Repetitive stress and microtrauma result in tendinosis and partial-thickness tears of the CET. The partial-thickness tears may subsequently become full-thickness tears.[2]
- Degeneration of the collagen fibrils, necrosis with hyaline and myxoid degeneration, angiofibroblastic proliferation, and scarring are the histological features of lateral epicondylitis.
- Tendinosis most commonly involves the deep layer of the CET, i.e. the ECRB tendon.[3]

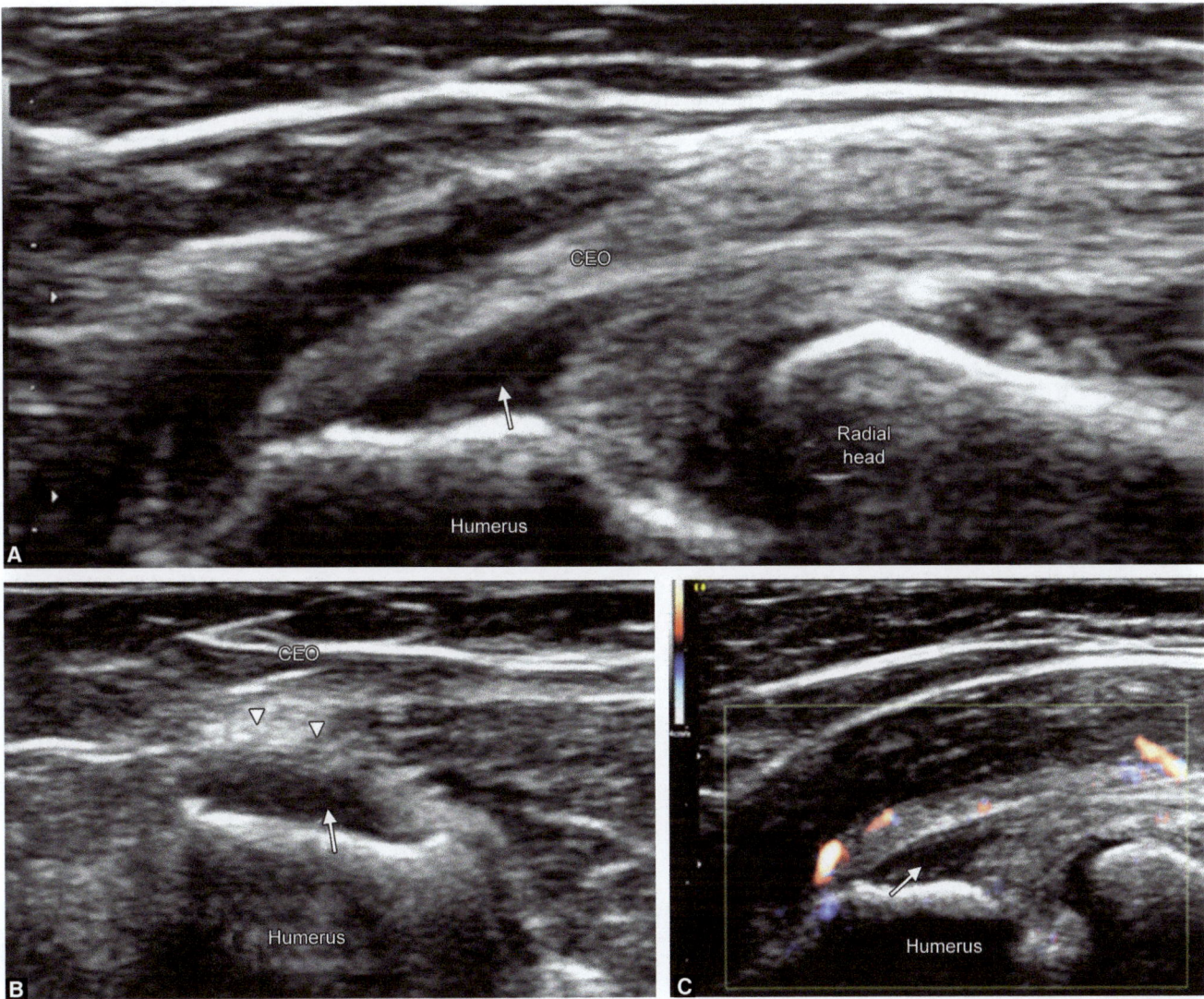

Figs. 2A to C: (A and B) Long axis and transverse images show a partial-thickness tear (arrow) involving middle and deep fibers of the common extensor origin (CEO); and (C) Power Doppler shows neovascularity in the CEO tendon suggesting active inflammation.

- *Ultrasound (US) findings in lateral epicondylitis*:
  - Tendon enlargement.
  - Tendinosis is seen as ill-defined or focal hypoechogenicity within the tendon along with loss of fibrillary pattern.
  - Tears are seen as hypoechoic or anechoic clefts with discontinuity of the tendon fibers (Figs. 1 and 2).
  - Intratendinous calcification.
  - Volume loss in the tendon is seen in chronic tendon tears.
  - Cortical irregularity and spur formation in the underlying lateral epicondyle.
  - Power Doppler may show increased flow in the presence of active inflammation as well as tendon healing.
- Role of US in lateral epicondylitis is to confirm the clinical diagnosis, assessing the severity of the disease, to rule other causes of lateral elbow pain, and provide image guidance of therapeutic interventions.
- Other common causes that mimic cause lateral elbow pain are posterior interosseous nerve (PIN) entrapment, chondromalacia involving the radiocapitellar joint, intra-articular loose body, and posterolateral rotatory instability.

■ REFERENCES

1. Bunata RE, Brown DS, Capelo R. Anatomic factors related to the cause of tennis elbow. J Bone Joint Surg Am. 2007;89:1955-63.
2. Nirschl RP, Pettrone FA. Lateral and medial epicondylitis. In: Morrey BF (Ed). Master techniques in orthopedic surgery: the elbow. New York: Raven; 1994. pp. 537-52.
3. Martinoli C, Bianchi S, Giovagnorio F, et al. Ultrasound of the elbow. Skeletal Radiol. 2001;30:605-14.

Case 21

Calcific Tendinosis Involving the Common Flexor Origin

CLINICAL HISTORY

A 54-year-old female having pain along the medial aspect of the elbow since 2 months.

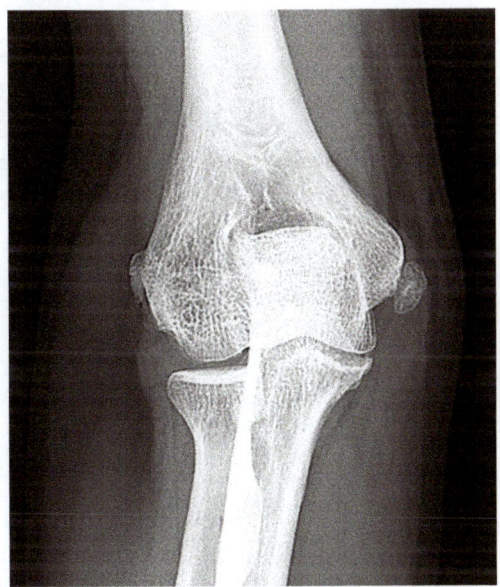

Fig. 1: Frontal radiograph of the elbow shows soft tissue calcification over the medial epicondyle. Enthesopathic changes are seen over the lateral epicondyle as well.

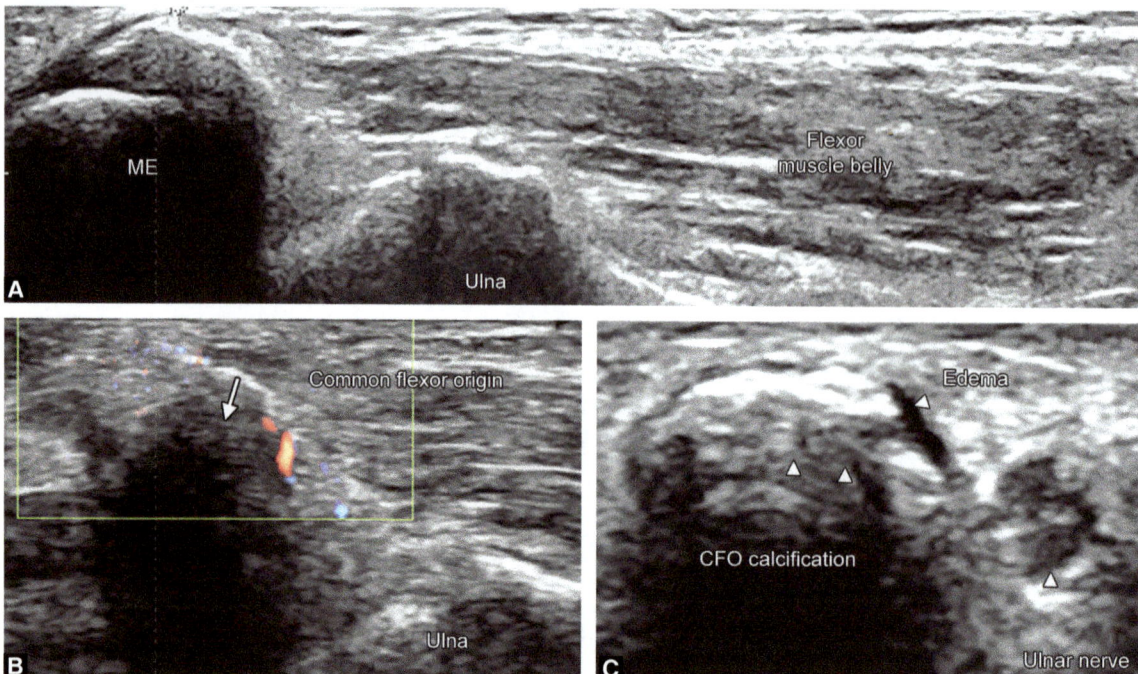

Figs. 2A to C: Long axis and transverse images show heterogeneous appearance of the peri-insertional fibers of the common flexor origin (CFO) along with nodular calcification (arrowheads and arrow) and edema. Power Doppler shows intratendinous neovascularity around the calcium.

■ DIAGNOSIS

Calcific tendinosis involving the common flexor origin of the elbow.

■ DISCUSSION

- Overuse injury at the site of origin of the common flexor tendon along the medial epicondyle of the humerus is referred to as medial epicondylitis. It is characterized by pain along the medial aspect of the elbow. This condition is also known as Golfer's elbow.
- The common flexor tendon along the medial aspect of the elbow is formed by the flexor carpi radialis (FCR), flexor carpi ulnaris (FCU), palmaris longus, and flexor digitorum superficialis (FDS) muscles.[1]
- The FCR and the pronator teres share a common origin from the anterior aspect of the medial epicondyle and are primarily involved in medial epicondylitis.[2]
- Valgus forces generated during the throwing phase result in stretching of the tendons leading to microtrauma.
- The anterior band of the ulnar collateral ligament (UCL) plays an important role in resisting valgus stress across the elbow joint.[3] Hence, UCL must be assessed during ultrasound (US) evaluation of medial epicondylitis.
- *Ultrasound findings in medial epicondylitis*:
    - Tendon enlargement. Fluid may be seen adjacent to the thickened tendon.
    - Heterogeneous echotexture of the tendon.
    - Intratendinous calcification.
    - Small tears are seen as hypoechoic regions within the tendon with tendon discontinuity.
- *Differential diagnosis of medial elbow pain*: Ulnar collateral ligament injury, ulnar neuritis, osteoarthritis, and posteromedial elbow impingement.

■ REFERENCES

1. Blease S, Stoller DW, Safran MR, et al. The elbow. In: Stoller DW (Ed). Magnetic resonance imaging in orthopaedics and sports medicine, 3rd edition. Philadelphia: Lippincott Williams & Wilkins; 2007. pp. 1463-626.
2. Faro F, Wolf JM. Lateral epicondylitis: review and current concepts. J Hand Surg Am. 2007;32:1271-9.
3. Nazarian LN, McShane JM, Ciccotti MG, et al. Dynamic US of the anterior band of the ulnar collateral ligament of the elbow in asymptomatic major league baseball pitchers. Radiology. 2003;227:149-54.

Case 22

Subcutaneous Rheumatoid Nodule

■ CLINICAL HISTORY

A 63-year-old female presented with progressively increasing painless swelling over the extensor aspect of the forearm since 8 months (Fig. 1). She is known to have rheumatoid arthritis since 21 years.

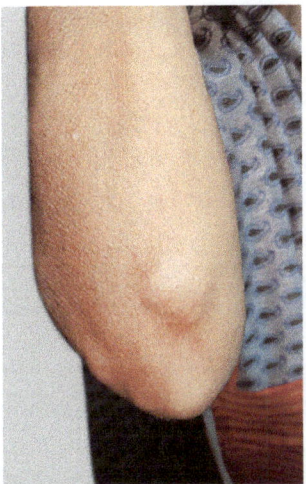

Fig. 1: Progressively enlarging painless nodule along the extensor aspect of forearm.

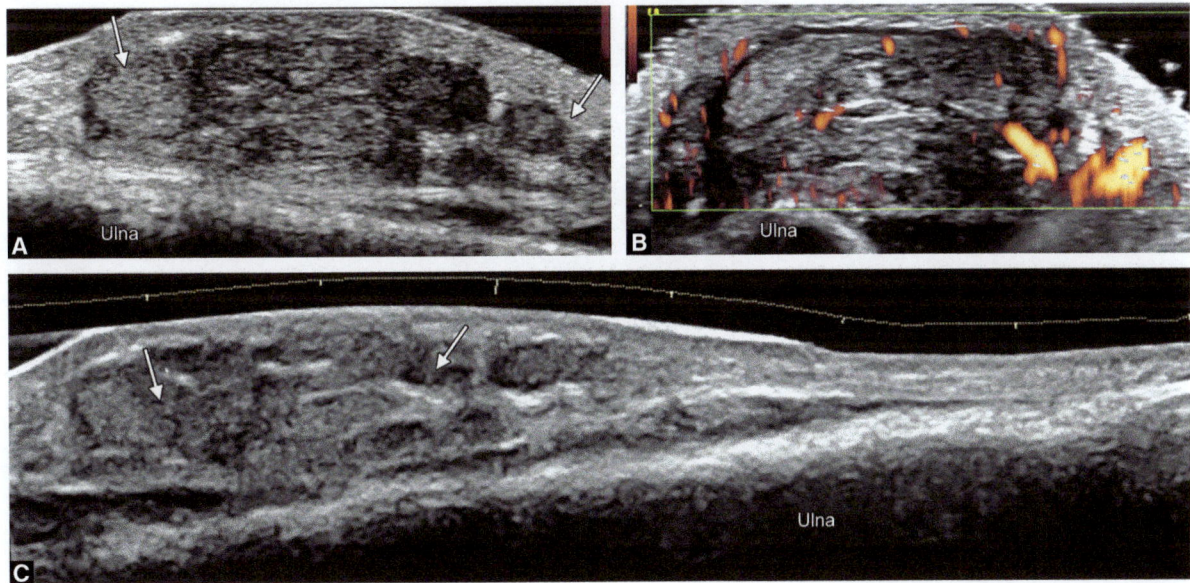

Figs. 2A to C: Long-axis (Figures A and C) and transverse (Figure B) images show an irregular isoechoic to hypoechoic solid lesion (arrows) in the subcutaneous fat without any evidence of erosion of the underlying cortex. Power Doppler shows neovascularity within the nodule.

■ DIAGNOSIS

Rheumatoid nodule.

■ DISCUSSION

- Subcutaneous rheumatoid nodules are seen in 20–30% of the patients with rheumatoid arthritis (RA).
- Pathologically, the rheumatoid nodules consist of central areas of necrosis surrounded by connective tissue.[1]
- Rheumatoid nodules are frequently encountered over osseous prominences that are repeatedly exposed to mechanical irritation. Common sites include extensor aspect of the forearm, calcaneum, heel, and the fingers.[2]
- On ultrasound, the nodules appear relatively homogeneous and mildly hypoechoic. Well-defined hypoechoic areas at the center of the lesion (Figs. 2A to C).
- Presence of intralesional vascularity (on power Doppler) depends on the disease activity.

■ REFERENCES

1. el-Noueam KI, Giuliano V, Schweitzer ME, et al. Rheumatoid nodules: MR/pathological correlation. J Comput Assist Tomogr. 1997;21:796-9.
2. Prete M, Racanelli V, Digiglio L, et al. Extra-articular manifestations of rheumatoid arthritis: an update. Autoimmun Rev. 2011;11:123-31.

Case 23

Chronic Partial-thickness Tear of the Triceps Muscle

■ CLINICAL HISTORY

A 27-year-old male presented with vague pain along the posteromedial aspect of the right elbow during extension of the elbow. He is a professional bodybuilder and gave history of anabolic steroid abuse.

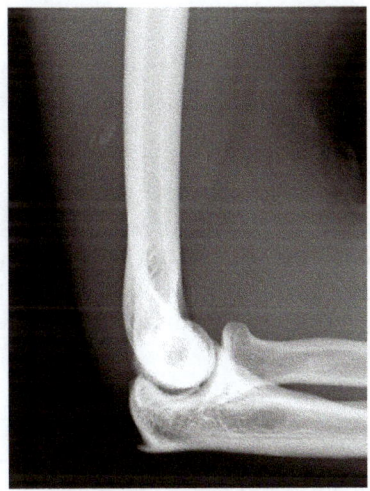

Fig. 1: Lateral radiograph of the elbow shows soft tissue calcification along the posterior aspect of the humerus.

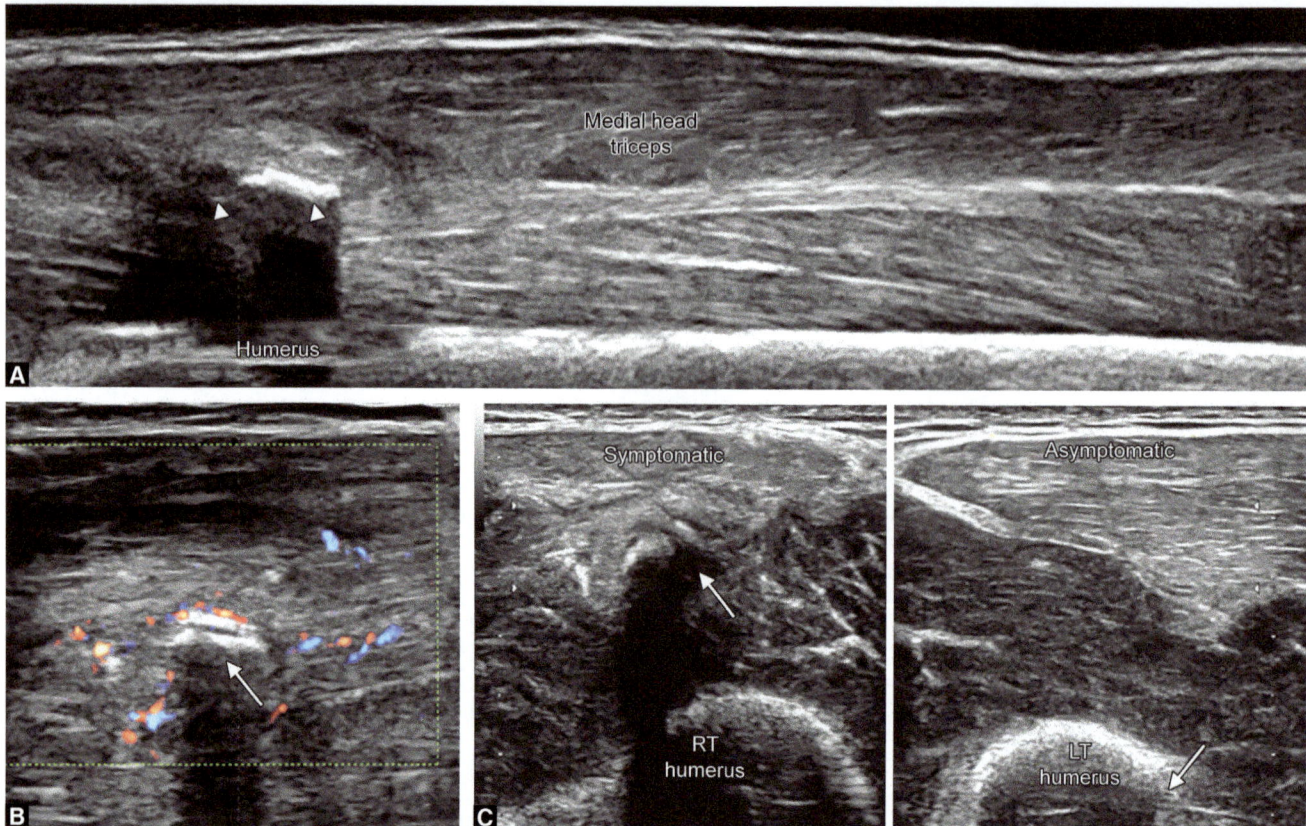

Figs. 2A to C: Long-axis (Figures A and B) and transverse (Figure C) images show a partial-thickness tear (arrowheads) at the myoaponeurotic junction of the medial head of triceps muscle belly. Calcification (arrows) is seen at the margins of the tear. Power Doppler (Figure B) shows neovascularity around the tear. Comparison with the asymptomatic side (Figure C) makes the heterogeneous appearance of the involved muscle more obvious pronounced. (RT: right; LT: left)

■ DIAGNOSIS

Chronic partial-thickness tear of the medial head of triceps muscle belly along the myoaponeurotic junction with calcification.

Case 24

Osseous Avulsion Injury of Triceps Tendon

■ CLINICAL HISTORY

A 62-year-old female presented an acute pain and swelling along the posterior aspect of the elbow following a fall.

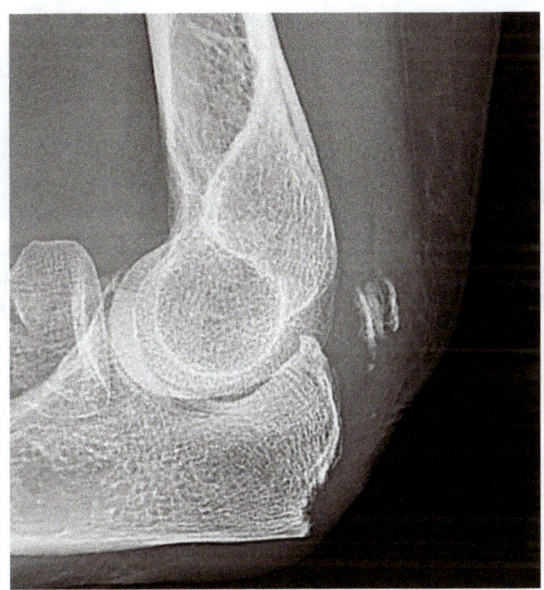

Fig. 1: Lateral radiograph of the elbow shows linear osseous flakes along the posterior aspect of the elbow joint. Focal cortical defect is seen over the olecranon process.

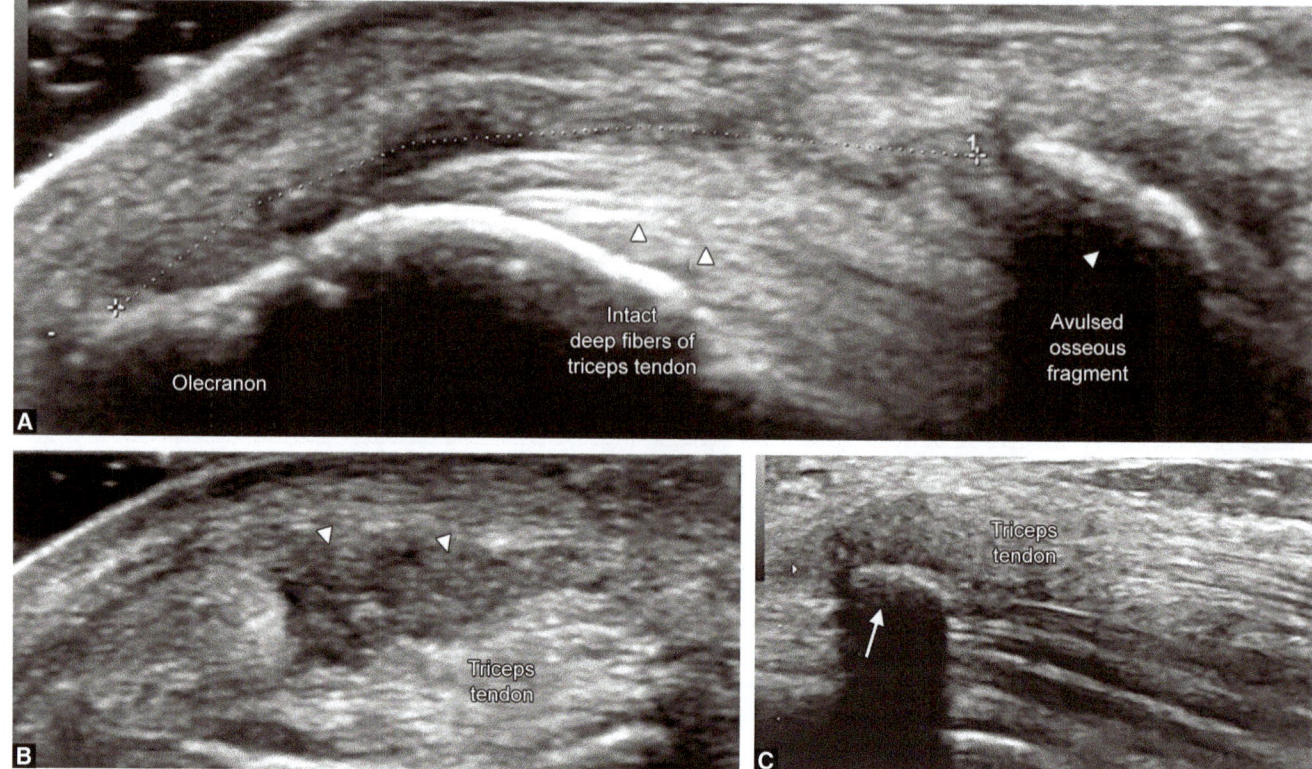

Figs. 2A to C: Long-axis (Figures A and C) and transverse (Figure B) images show a partial-thickness osseous avulsion injury of triceps tendon at its olecranon insertion. The avulsed osseous fragment (arrow) is seen as a hyperechoic structure with distal shadowing within the retracted tendon fibers (Figure A). Transverse image (Figure B) shows the triceps tendon tear (arrowheads) that shows involvement of the posterior fibers.

■ DIAGNOSIS

Partial-thickness osseous avulsion injury involving the posterior third of triceps tendon (lateral and long heads).

Case 25

Distal Biceps Tendon Tear

CLINICAL HISTORY

A 45-year-old male presented with acute pain and swelling along the anterior aspect of the proximal forearm, while working out in the gymnasium.

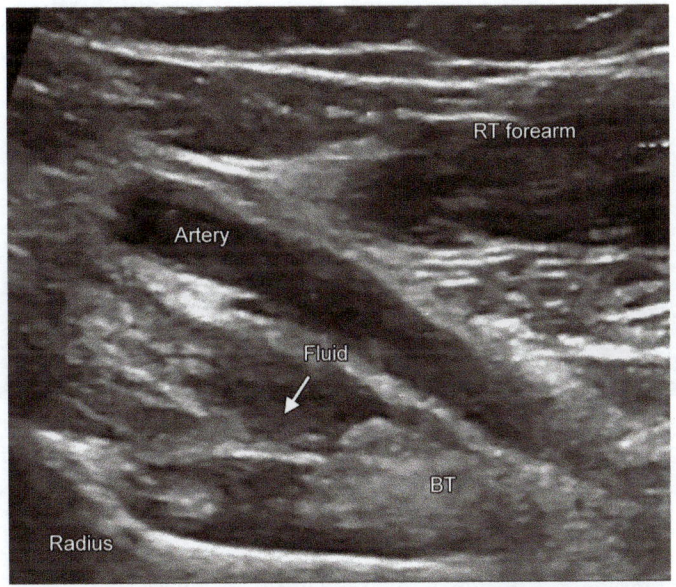

Fig. 1: Long-axis image shows a full-thickness tear (arrow) in the distal biceps tendon. (BT: biceps tendon; RT: right)

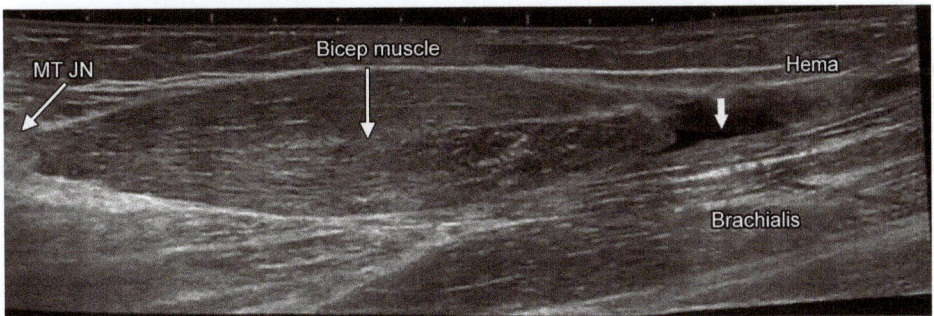

Fig. 2: Long-axis extended field of view shows a full-thickness tear (thick arrow) in the distal biceps tendon. The defect is filled with a hematoma. (MT JN: Proximal myotendinous junction)

DIAGNOSIS

Full-thickness tear of the distal biceps tendon with proximal retraction of the torn margins.

Case 26

Partial-thickness Tear of the Ulnar Collateral Ligament of the Elbow

■ CLINICAL HISTORY

A 38-year-old male presented with pain along the medial aspect of the left elbow following a fall from the bike. The pain is aggravated while performing activities that cause valgus strain on the elbow.

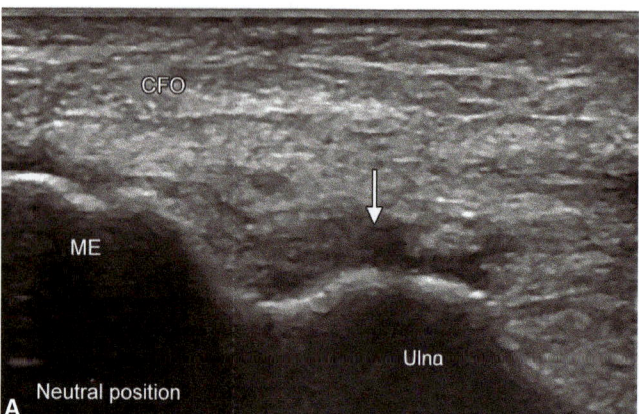 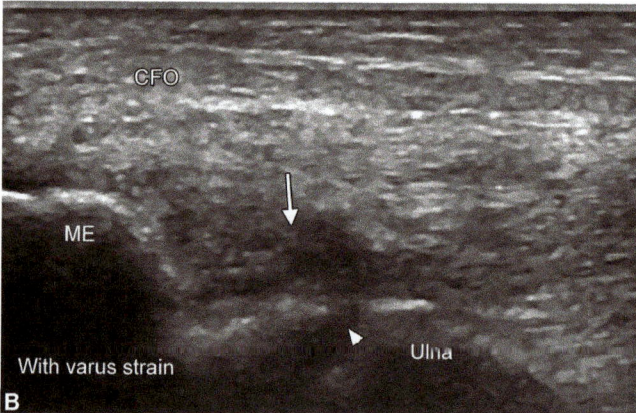

Figs. 1A and B: Long-axis images of the ulnar collateral ligament show discontinuity of the fibers of the anterior band, suggestive of a full-thickness tear (arrows). Imaging of the elbow with various strain shows mild widening of the medial joint space (arrowhead) of the elbow. (CFO: common flexor origin; ME: medial epicondyle)

■ DIAGNOSIS

Full-thickness tear of the anterior band of the ulnar collateral ligament (UCL).

■ DISCUSSION

- During varus stress, the UCL functions as a medial stabilizer of the elbow joint.
- The UCL consists of three bundles: (1) anterior, (2) posterior, and (3) transverse. The anterior bundle is the strongest component of the UCL and is functionally the most important.[1]
- *Mechanism of UCL injuries*:
  - Acute or chronic repetitive overstretching of the elbow in valgus stress during the acceleration phase of throwing.
  - Fall or posterior dislocation of the elbow joint.
- *Ultrasound (US) features of UCL injury*:
  - Thickened hypoechoic MCL with surrounding edema
  - Calcification
  - Discontinuity of fibers
  - Osseous avulsion injury
  - Dynamic scans with valgus stress show widening of the ulnotrochlear joint space.

■ REFERENCE

1. Morrey BF, An KN. Articular and ligamentous contributions to the stability of the elbow joint. Am J Sports Med. 1983;11:315-9.

Case 27

Myositis Ossificans

■ CLINICAL HISTORY

A 14-year-old male presented with a progressively enlarging firm lump along the medial aspect of the elbow since 1 month. The patient gave a history of falling on an outstretched hand, 2 months ago.

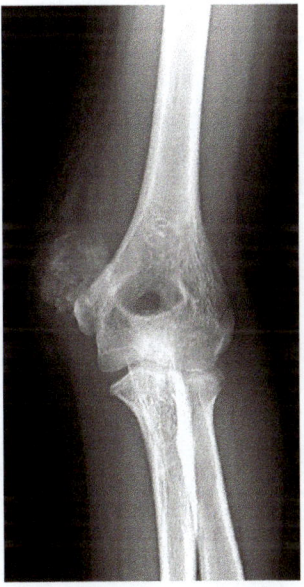

Fig. 1: Frontal radiograph of the elbow shows well-defined periarticular soft tissue calcification along the medial aspect.

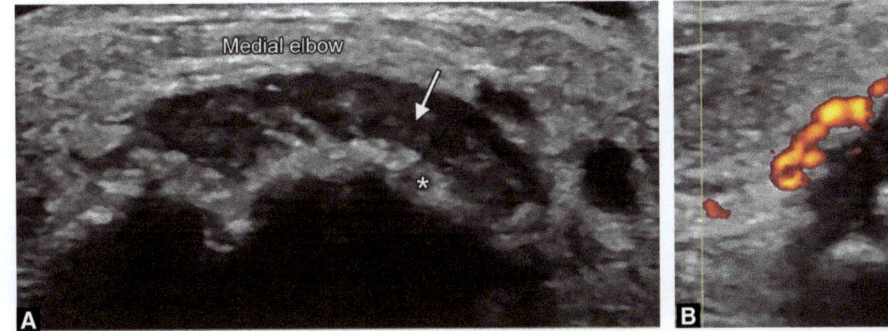

Figs. 2A and B: (A) Transverse image along the medial aspect of the elbow shows an infiltrative intramuscular lesion demonstrating a peripheral hypoechoic rim (arrow) surrounding a hyperechoic zone of calcification(*); and (B) Another hypoechoic zone (arrowhead) is seen deeper to the hyperechoic zone of calcification. Power Doppler shows hyperemia at the periphery of the lesion.

■ DIAGNOSIS

Myositis ossificans (MO).

■ DISCUSSION

- Myositis ossificans is an intramuscular self-limiting benign lesion, which may be regarded as an inflammatory pseudotumor.
- Although MO is considered to occur as a sequelae of blunt trauma to the muscle, quite often there is no history of any obvious injury.[1]
- Histologically, the MO demonstrates a zonal phenomenon where three distinct zones are observed. The inner zone consists of hemorrhage, fibroblasts, and necrotic muscle tissue. The middle zone is made up of immature osteoid and foci of cartilage. Mature bone forms the outer zone.
- Ultrasound (US) findings of MO depend upon the age of the lesion and evolving the histopathological features.
- More commonly, MO demonstrates a zonal appearance on US. A hypoechoic band encircling an echogenic rim is seen. Another hypoechoic zone may be seen deep to the echogenic rim. As the duration from the primary insult increases, the peripheral hypoechoic rim becomes more echogenic as calcification occurs in this zone (Figs. 2A and B).
- It is advisable to correlate the US findings with the radiographic findings.

■ REFERENCE

1. Nuovo MA, Norman A, Chumas J, et al. Myositis ossificans with atypical clinical, radiographic, or pathologic findings: a review of 23 cases. Skeletal Radiol. 1992;21:87-101.

Case 28

Volar Wrist Ganglion

■ CLINICAL HISTORY

A 37-year-old woman presented with multiple painless nodules along the volar aspect of the wrist.

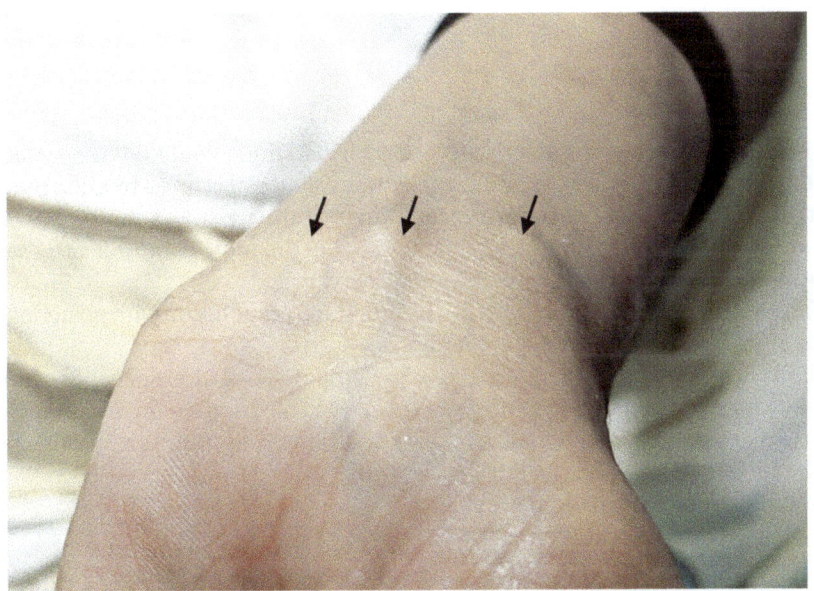

Fig. 1: Multiple painless nodules along the volar aspect of the wrist.

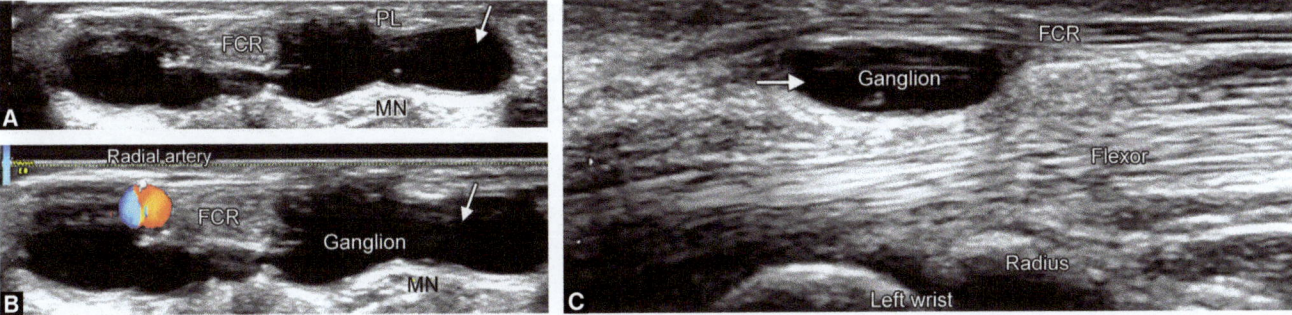

Figs. 2A to C: Short-axis (Figures A and B) and long-axis (Figure C) images show a lobulated anechoic ganglion along the volar aspect of the wrist. The flexor carpi radialis (FCR) and the palmaris longus (PL) tendons lie over the ganglion and are seen to indent it. The radial artery is seen closely abutting the ganglion. (MN: Median nerve)

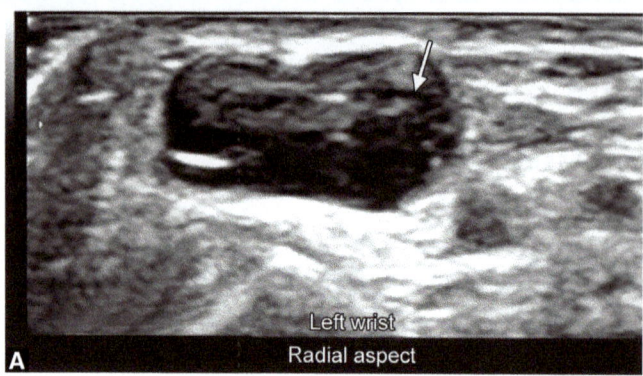 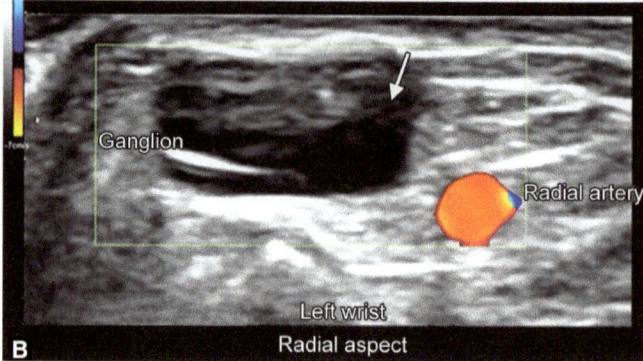

Figs. 3A and B: Short-axis images show a ganglion (arrows) at the radial aspect of the wrist along the volar surface. The radial artery is seen along the ulnar aspect of the ganglion.

■ DIAGNOSIS

Ganglion.

■ DISCUSSION

- A ganglion is a periarticular benign cystic soft tissue lesion formed due to mucoid degeneration of the joint capsule, tendon sheath, or the tendon. The lesion containing gelatinous material is lined by collagen.
- Ganglia are most the most commonly occurring focal lesions of the wrist and hand.[1] 60–70% of the ganglia occur along the dorsum of the wrist—the scapholunate ligament being the most common site. Quite often, a pedicle may be visualized communicating the ganglion with the joint cavity.
- On ultrasound (US), a simple ganglion is visualized as a well-defined cystic lesion with posterior acoustic enhancement.[2] The lesion is devoid of vascularity on Power Doppler images.
- Complex cystic ganglia may show thickened walls, locules, and low-level internal echoes (due to mucin).
- A collapsed ganglion with synovial hypertrophy may appear as a solid nodule on US, mimicking a soft tissue tumor.
- During US evaluation of a volar wrist ganglion (Fig. 1), it is important to describe its relationship with the flexor tendons, radial artery, and the median nerve (Figs. 2 and 3).[3]
- Ultrasound-guided drainage of a ganglion may be done.

■ REFERENCES

1. Athanasian EA. Bone and soft tissue tumors. In: Green DP, Hotchkiss RN, Pederson WC, Wolfe SW (Eds). Green's operative hand surgery, 5th edition. Philadelphia: Churchill Livingstone; 2005. pp. 2221-32.
2. Bianchi S, Abdelwahab IF, Zwass A, et al. Ultrasonographic evaluation of wrist ganglia. Skeletal Radiol. 1994;23:201-3.
3. Wright TW, Cooney WP, Ilstrup M. Anterior wrist ganglion. J Hand Surg. 1994;19:954-8.

Case 29

Carpal Tunnel Syndrome

CLINICAL HISTORY

A 47-year-old woman presented with pain and vague tingling sensation along the first four fingers.

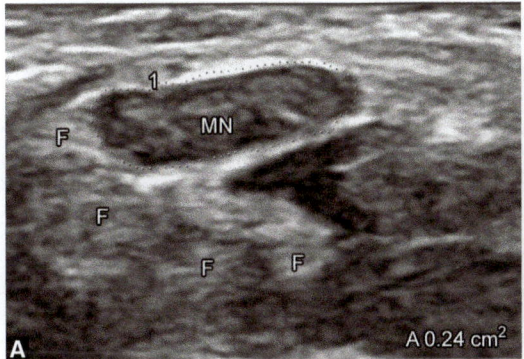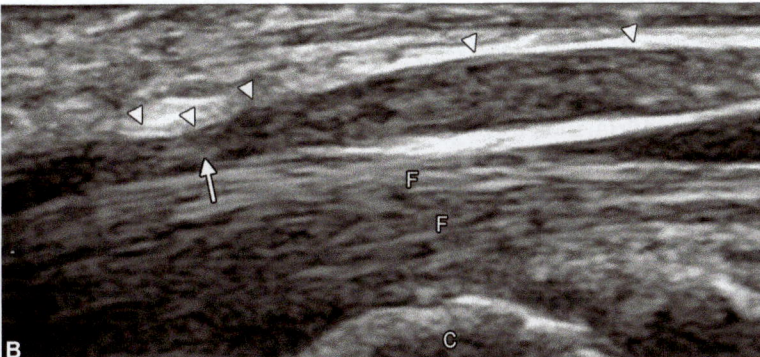

Figs. 1A and B: (A) Short-axis image shows an increase in the cross-sectional area of the median nerve (MN). The flexor tendons (F) are seen as echogenic rounded structures on the short-axis image; (B) Long-axis image shows flattening (arrow) of the thickened median nerve (arrowheads) as it enters the carpal tunnel. (C: carpal bone)

DIAGNOSIS

Compressive neuropathy of the median nerve (MN) carpal tunnel syndrome (CTS).

DISCUSSION

- Carpal tunnel is a fibro-osseous tunnel at the wrist joint bounded by the flexor retinaculum along the volar aspect and carpal bones along the dorsal aspect. As the MN traverses the wrist joint, the carpal tunnel is a potential site of MN entrapment. The compressive neuropathy is referred as CTS. CTS is the most commonly encountered nerve entrapment syndrome of the upper limb.
- *Predisposing factors for CTS*: Systemic neuropathies, diabetes mellitus, pregnancy, hypothyroidism, amyloidosis, and space-occupying lesions within the carpal tunnel.
- Median nerve compression results in pain or tingling sensation along the area of MN distribution—typically seen along the thumb, index finger, middle finger, and radial half of the ring finger.
- Diagnosis of CTS is primarily based on clinical examination and nerve conduction studies.
- Normal appearance of the MN on ultrasound (US) scan does not rule out CTS.
- *Role of ultrasound in CTS*:
    - To assess the morphology of MN.
    - Quantification of the MN enlargement and compression.
    - To identify space-occupying lesions within the carpal tunnel that result in MN compression.
    - When nerve conduction tests have equivocal results.

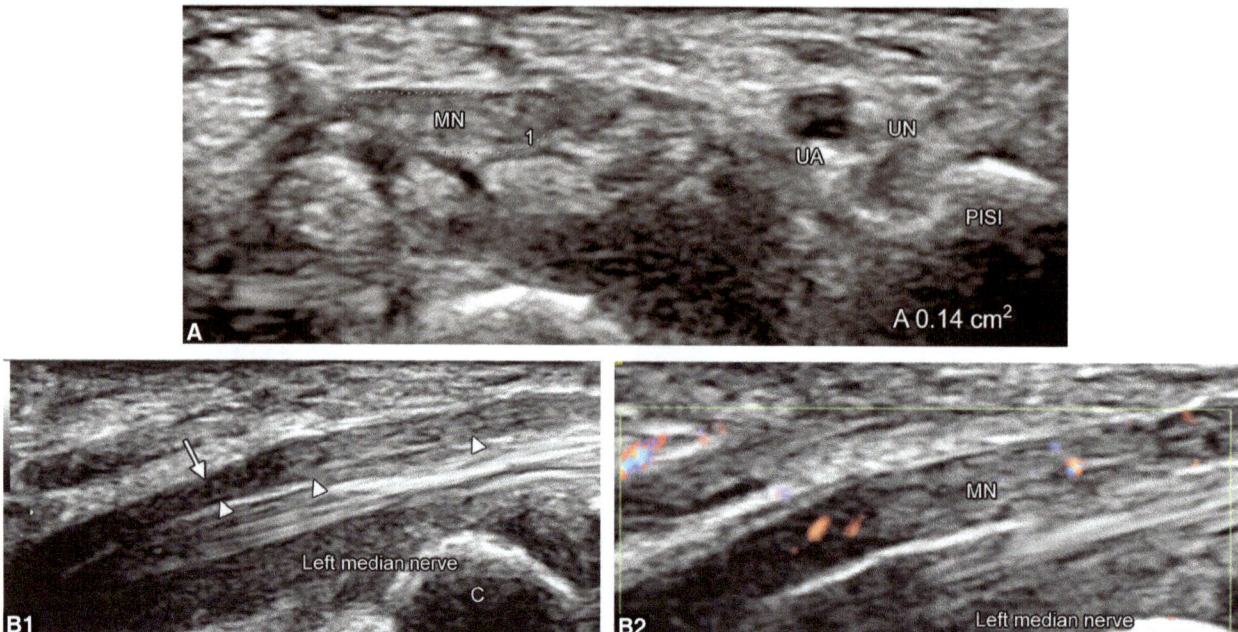

Figs. 2A and B: (A) Short-axis image shows an increase in the cross-sectional area of the median nerve (MN). (B1 and B2) Long-axis image (Figure B1) shows flattening (arrow) of the median nerve (arrowheads) as it enters the carpal tunnel. Figure B2 shows intraneural vascularity within the median nerve (MN). (C: carpal bone; PISI: pisiform bone; UA: ulnar artery; UN: ulnar nerve)

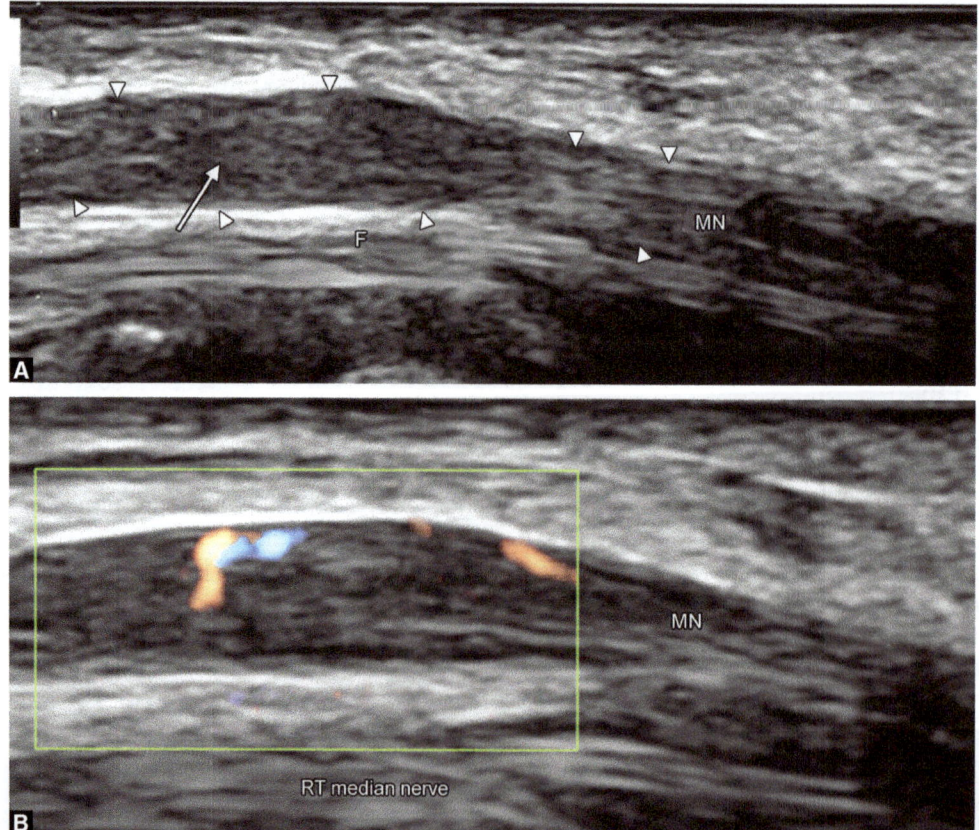

Figs. 3A and B: (A) Long-axis image shows flattening (arrowheads) of the thickened median nerve (MN) as it enters the carpal tunnel. The nerve proximal to the carpal tunnel appears edematous (arrow) and shows loss of normal echotexture. (B) Intraneural vascularity within the MN. (F: flexor tendon; RT: right)

- *Ultrasound findings in CTS*:
    - The compressed MN appears enlarged and hypoechoic in the proximal tunnel and flattened in the distal half of the carpal tunnel. The sudden change in the caliber of the MN is known as a "notch sign" (Figs. 1B and 2B).
    - The MN is considered to be thickened when the cross-sectional area (CSA) is more than 10 mm^2. Some authors consider 12 mm^2 as a cutoff for normal CSA of the MN. The CSA of the MN is calculated at the level of pisiform bone.[1]
    - Quantification of MN thickening may be done by measuring the nerve at two levels, i.e. at the distal forearm (using pronator quadratus as the landmark) and at the wrist joint (at the level of pisiform). A difference of CSA of more than 2 mm^2 is considered significant.[2]
    - Hypoechoic appearance of the MN along with loss of fascicular pattern (Figs. 2B and 3A).[1]
    - Intraneural hypervascularity on color Doppler (Figs. 2B, 3A and B).
    - Palmar bowing of the flexor retinaculum by more than 2 mm. The flexor retinaculum is assessed at the level of distal carpal tunnel (hamate-trapezium level).
    - *Additional space-occupying lesions*: Tenosynovitis, ganglion cysts, anomalous muscles, persistent median artery, and callus.

REFERENCES

1. Duncan I, Sullivan P, Lomas F. Sonography in the diagnosis of carpal tunnel syndrome. AJR Am J Roentgenol. 1999;173:681-4.
2. Klauser AS, Halpern EJ, De Zordo, T, et al. Carpal tunnel syndrome assessment with US: value of additional cross-sectional area measurements of the median nerve in patients versus healthy volunteers. Radiology. 2009;250:171-7.

CASE 30

Fibrolipomatous Hamartoma of the Median Nerve

■ CLINICAL HISTORY

A 36-year-old woman presented with an ill-defined fullness along the volar aspect of the wrist. She gave a history of vague tingling sensation along the first four fingers.

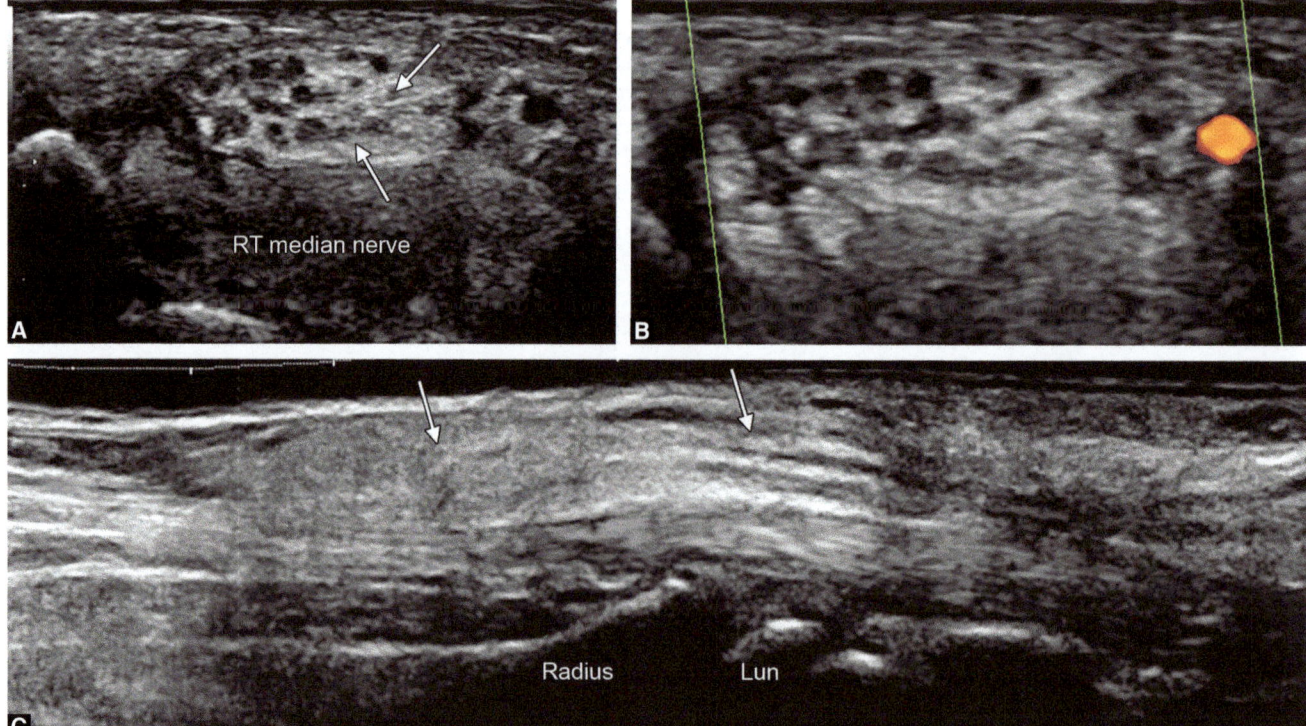

Figs. 1A to C: Short-axis (Figures A and B) and long-axis (Figure C) images show diffuse enlargement of the median nerve (arrows) along with a heterogeneous echotexture. On the short-axis images, the nerve fascicles appear thickened and are separated by echogenic soft tissue. Power Doppler does not show any significant intraneural vascularity. (Lun: lunate; RT: right)

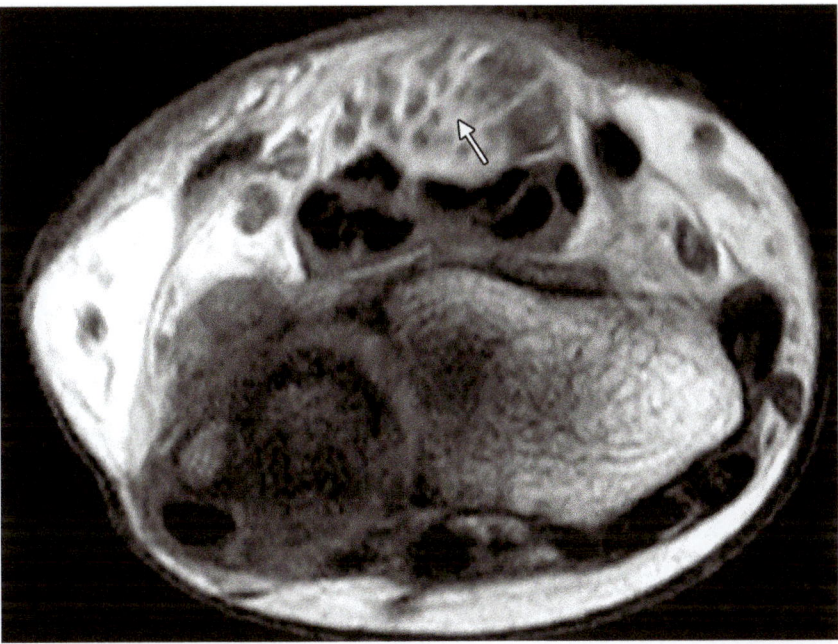

Fig. 2: T1-weighted axial image shows diffuse enlargement of the median nerve along fat separating the nerve fascicles.

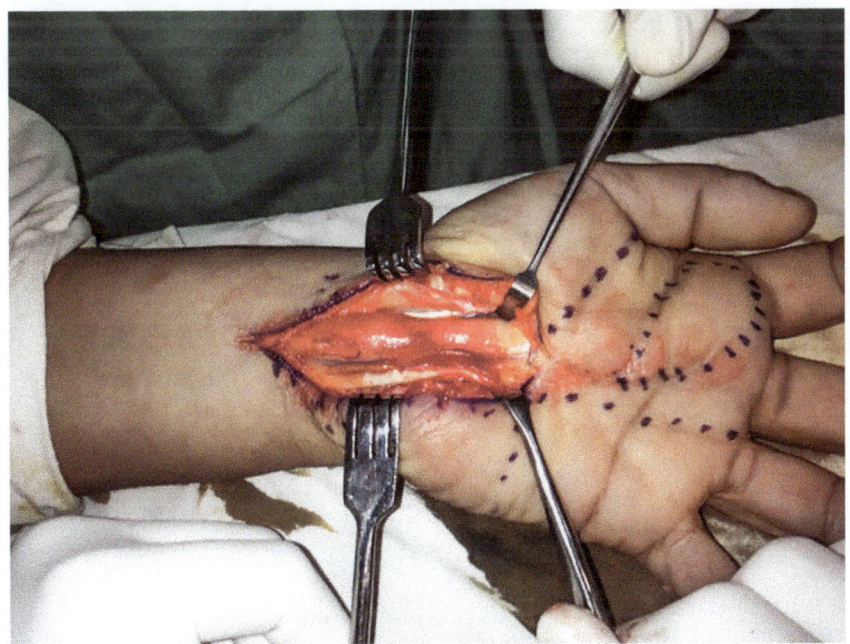

Fig. 3: Intraoperative appearance of the enlarged median nerve.

■ DIAGNOSIS

Fibrolipomatous hamartoma of the median nerve.

■ DISCUSSION

- Fibrolipomatous hamartoma is considered a developmental disorder caused due to hypertrophy of the mature fat and fibroblasts in the epineurium of the nerves.
- This entity is also known as fibrolipoma, perineural lipoma, and lipofibroma.
- Median nerve and its branches are most commonly affected.
- *Ultrasound (US) findings*:
    - Fusiform enlargement of the nerve in the distal forearm and wrist.
    - Increased volume of echogenic fat between the nerve fascicles.
    - Compression of the nerve at the carpal tunnel may cause the fascicles to appear hypoechoic and enlarged.

Case 31

Peripheral Nerve Sheath Tumor of the Median Nerve

■ CLINICAL HISTORY

A 42-year-old woman presented with a painful swelling along the volar aspect of wrist.

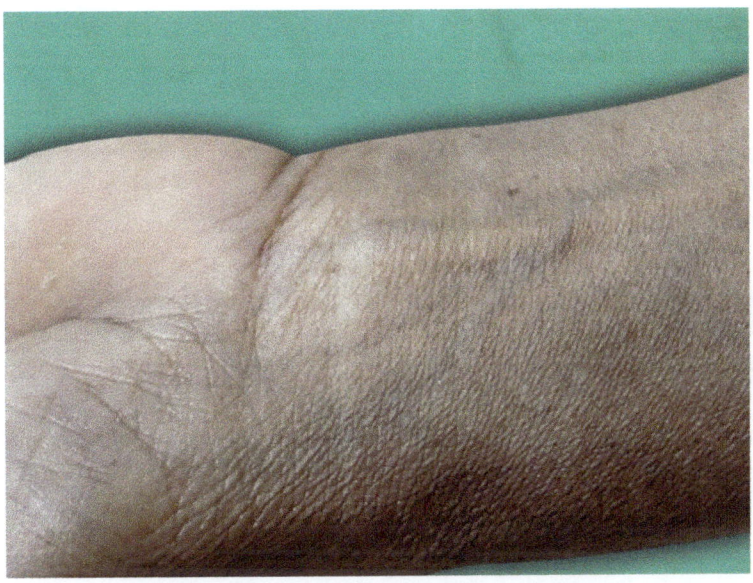

Fig. 1: Painful nodule along the volar aspect of wrist.

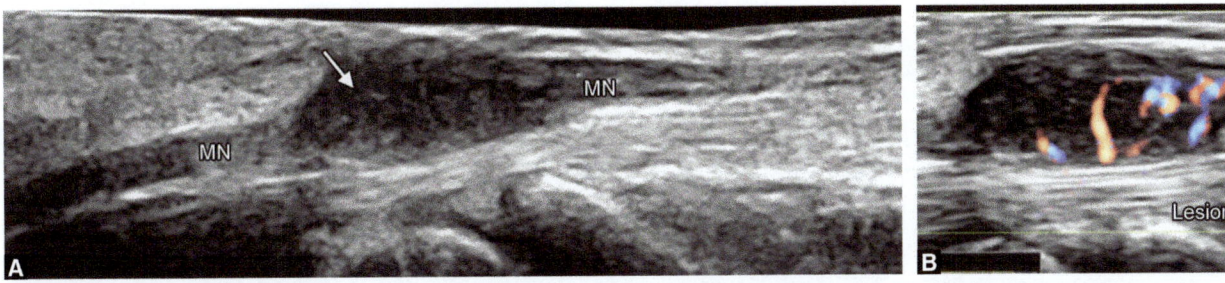

Figs. 2A and B: (A) Long-axis image shows a hypoechoic solid lesion (arrow) along the course of the median nerve (MN). The nerve is seen to enter and exit the lesion; and (B) Power Doppler shows marked intralesional vascularity.

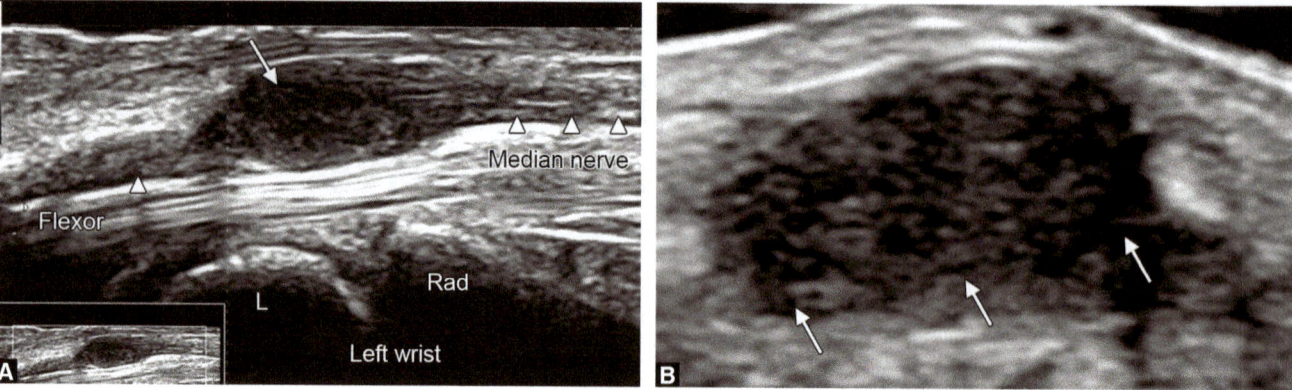

Figs. 3A and B: (A) Long-axis image shows a hypoechoic solid lesion (arrow) along the course of the median nerve (arrowheads); and (B) Short-axis image shows a solid hypoechoic lesion (arrows) in continuity with the nerve. (Rad: Radius)

◼ DIAGNOSIS

Peripheral nerve sheath tumor of the median nerve.

◼ DISCUSSION

- Primarily, there are two types of benign peripheral nerve sheath tumors—(1) schwannoma, and (2) neurofibroma.
- Schwannomas are slow growing tumors arising from Schwann cells. They are eccentrically located with respect to the nerve and do not contain axons.
- Neurofibromas are closely related to the nerve. On histopathology, there is a predominance of perineural cells.
- Morphologically, neurofibromas are classified as localized (most common), diffuse, and plexiform types.
- *Ultrasound findings of peripheral nerve sheath tumors*:
    - Hypoechoic solid lesions. Neurofibromas tend to be more fusiform.
    - While schwannomas are located at the periphery of the nerve, the neurofibromas seem to be intimately related to the nerve. The lesion is visualized along the course of a nerve. On the long-axis images, a nerve may be seen entering and exiting the lesion.
    - Intralesional cysts may be seen when there is accumulation of myxoid matrix.
    - Schwannomas appear as hypervascular lesions of color and power Doppler.

Case 32

Tenosynovitis of the Flexor Tendon Sheath at the Wrist Joint

CLINICAL HISTORY

A 36-year-old woman presented with a tingling numbness in her hand. She is a known case of rheumatoid arthritis.

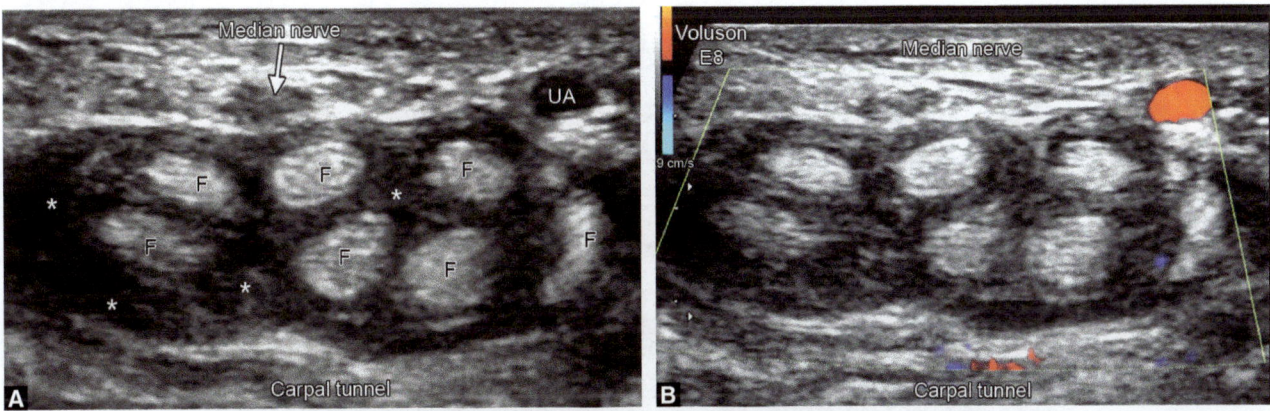

Figs. 1A and B: (A) Transverse images show diffuse synovial thickening (asterisks) within the flexor tendon sheath at the level of carpal tunnel. The median nerve (arrow) is located above the flexor tendon sheath; (B) Color Doppler does not show any significant vascularity within the thickened synovium. (F: flexor tendons; UA: ulnar artery)

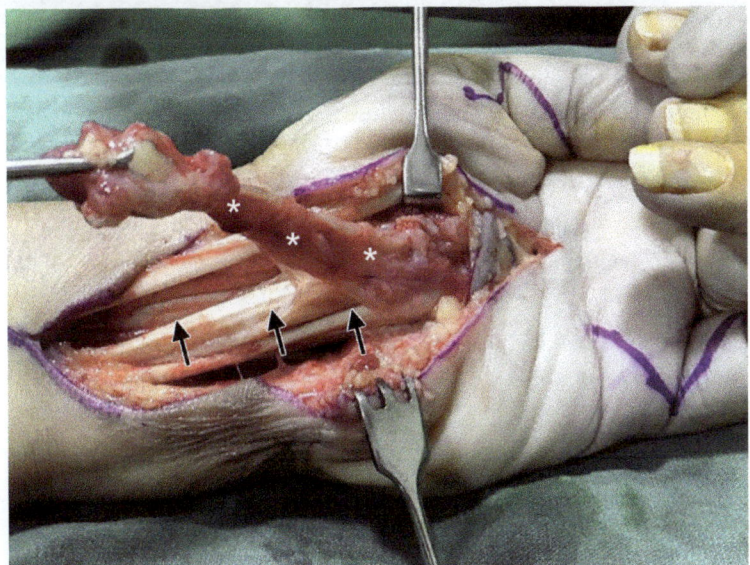

Fig. 2: Intraoperative image. Synovial thickening (asterisks). Flexor tendons (black arrows).

DIAGNOSIS

Tenosynovitis of the flexor tendon sheath resulting in secondary compression of the median nerve.

CASE 33

De Quervain's Tenosynovitis

■ CLINICAL HISTORY

A 28-year-old woman (chef by occupation) presented with pain along the radial aspect of the wrist.

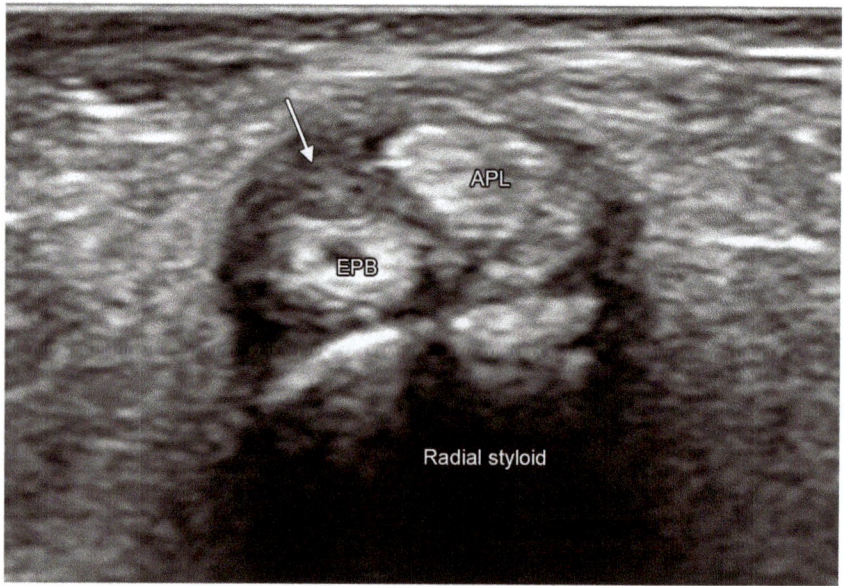

Fig. 1: Transverse image at the level of radial styloid shows diffuse thickening of the tendon sheath (arrow) along the extensor compartment I tendons. (APL: abductor pollicis longus; EPB: extensor pollicis brevis)

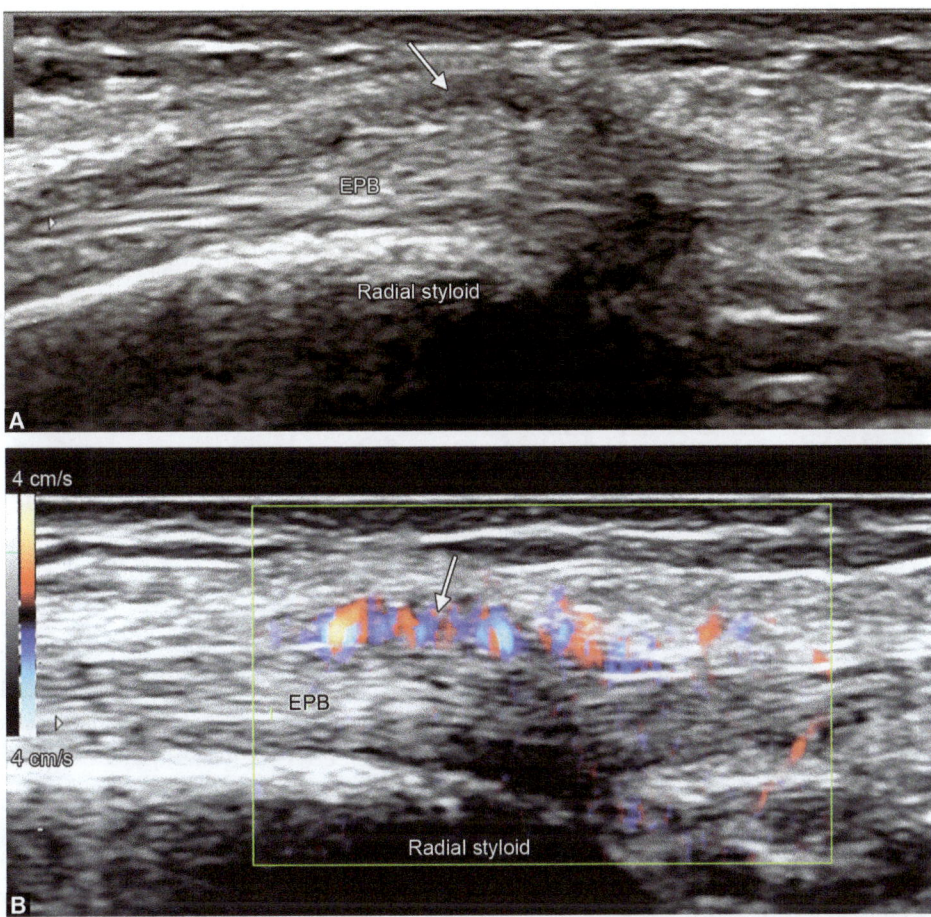

Figs. 2A and B: (A) Long-axis image at the level of radial styloid shows diffuse thickening of the tendon sheath (arrow) along the extensor compartment I tendons. The extensor pollicis brevis (EPB) tendon shows normal fibrillary pattern; and (B) Long-axis image with power Doppler shows increased vascularity in the thickened tendon sheath.

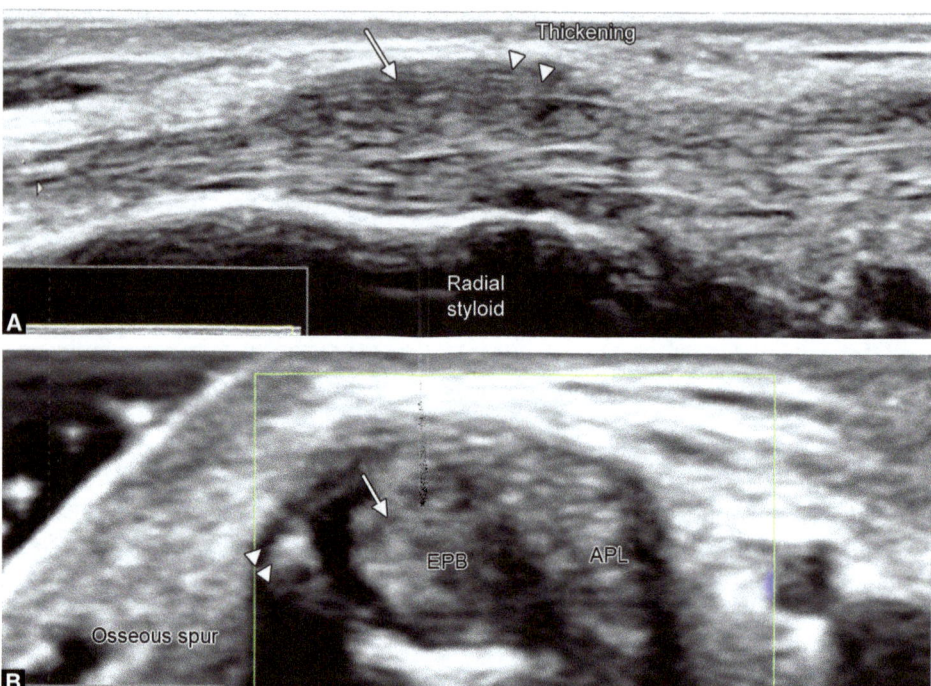

Figs. 3A and B: Long-axis (A) and transverse (B) images show mild fluid in the extensor compartment I tendon sheath along with thickening (arrow) of the extensor pollicis brevis (EPB) tendon. Figure B shows an osseous spur (arrowheads) along the dorsal radial cortex. (APL: abductor pollicis longus)

DIAGNOSIS

Tenosynovitis involving the tendon sheath of extensor compartment I (De Quervain's tenosynovitis).

DISCUSSION

- Two tendons occupy the first extensor compartment of the wrist—(1) abductor pollicis longus (APL), and (2) extensor pollicis brevis (EPB).
- De Quervain's tenosynovitis is an overuse injury due to repeated extension and flexion of the wrist with an abducted thumb.
- The patient typically complains of pain over the radial styloid.
- Although De Quervain's disease is a clinical diagnosis, ultrasound (US) imaging can help in assessing the extent and severity of the tendon sheath inflammation, assess the integrity of tendons, and identify any other pathology that may mimic the disease.
- *Role of US in De Quervain's tenosynovitis*:
  - Enlarged and hypoechoic tendons with increased cross-sectional area. Interstitial tears of the tendon may be seen in chronic cases.
  - Effusion in the tendon sheath.
  - Thickened extensor retinaculum (Figs. 3A and B).
  - Detection of anatomical variants like accessory septae, multiple slips of the APL tendon.
  - Volar subluxation of extensor compartment I tendon may be identified as a postsurgical complication.

CASE 34

Attritional Tear of Extensor Tendon at the Wrist due to Chronic Impingement

■ CLINICAL HISTORY

A 67-year-old woman presented with inability to extend her index finger. She had undergone internal fixation for a fracture involving the lower end of radius.

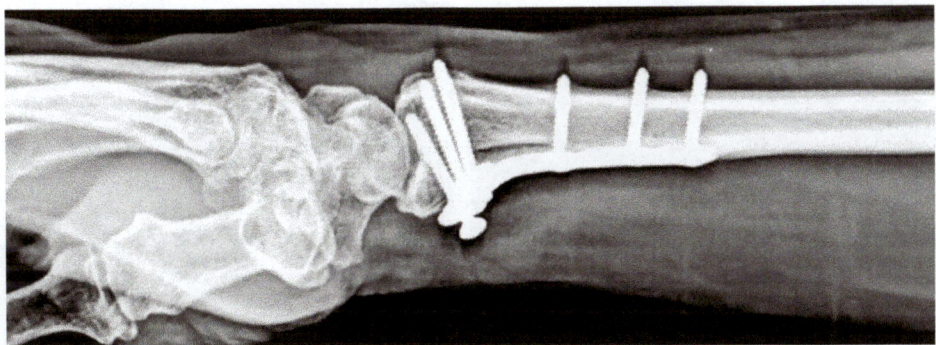

Fig. 1: Lateral radiograph of the wrist shows proud screws along the dorsal cortex of the distal radius.

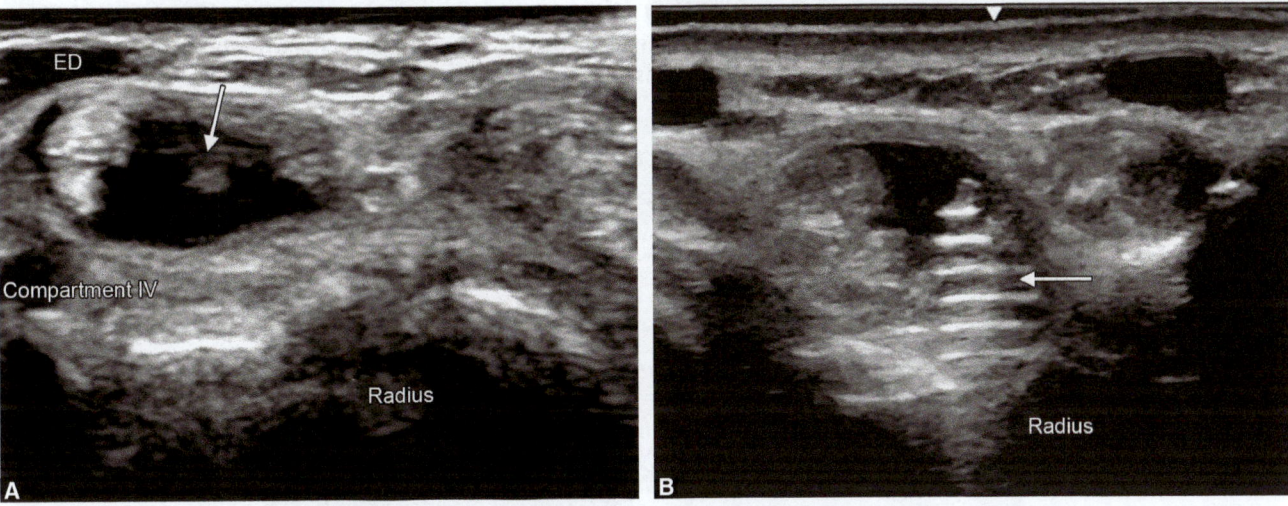

Figs. 2A and B: (A) Transverse image shows a tear (arrow) in the extensor compartment IV tendon. Fluid is seen within the defect; and (B) A proud screw jutting into the extensor compartment IV tendon sheath (arrow).

■ DIAGNOSIS

Attritional tear of extensor compartment IV tendon caused due to chronic impingement by a protruding screw.

Case 35

Inflammatory Tenosynovitis of Extensor Compartment IV Tendon Sheath at the Wrist Joint

■ CLINICAL HISTORY

A 22-year-old male presented with swelling along the dorsum of the right wrist. He is a known case of ankylosing spondylitis.

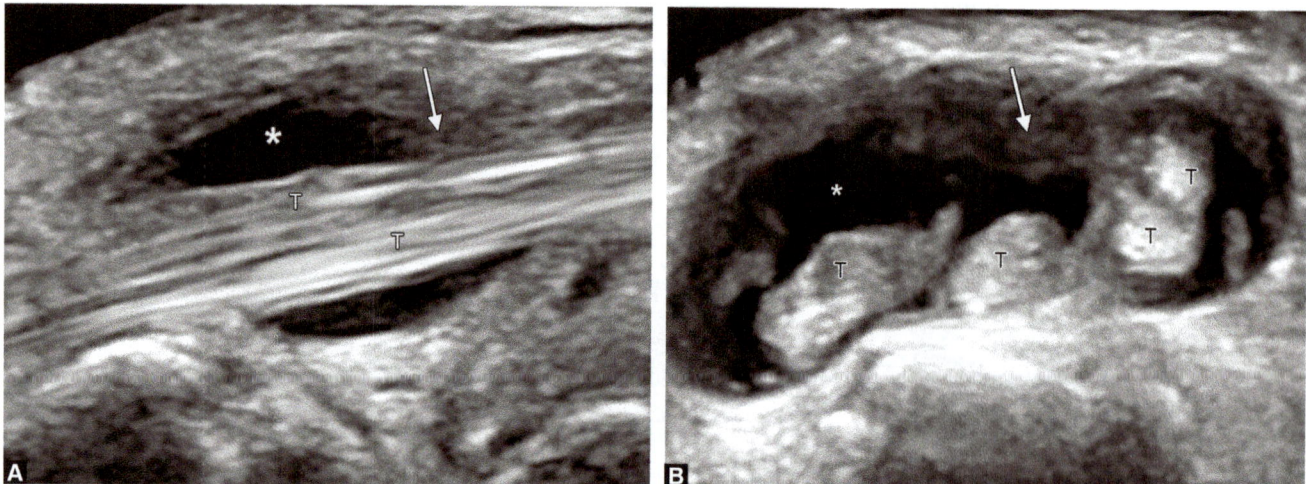

Figs. 1A and B: Long-axis (Figure A) and transverse (Figure B) images along the dorsal aspect of the wrist show effusion (*) and synovial hypertrophy (arrows) within the extensor compartment IV tendon sheath. (T: tendon)

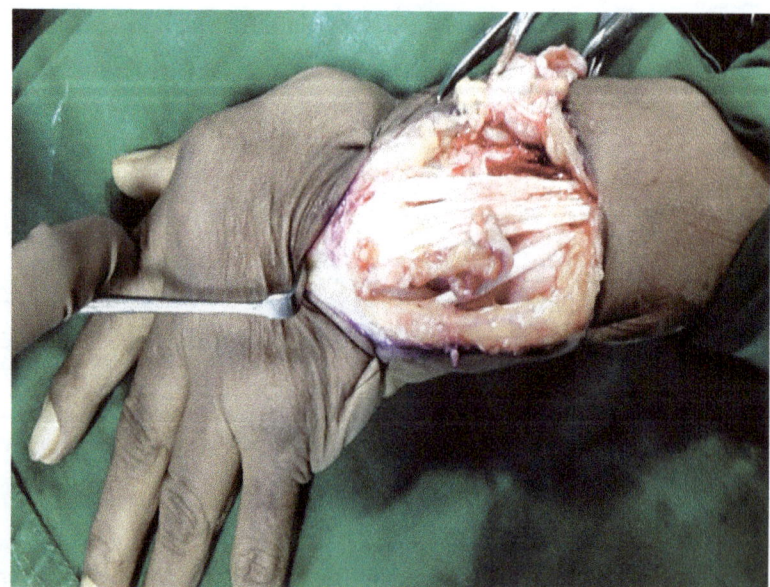

Fig. 2: Intraoperative picture shows thickened synovium over the extensor tendons.

DIAGNOSIS

Tenosynovitis involving the tendon sheath of extensor compartment IV.

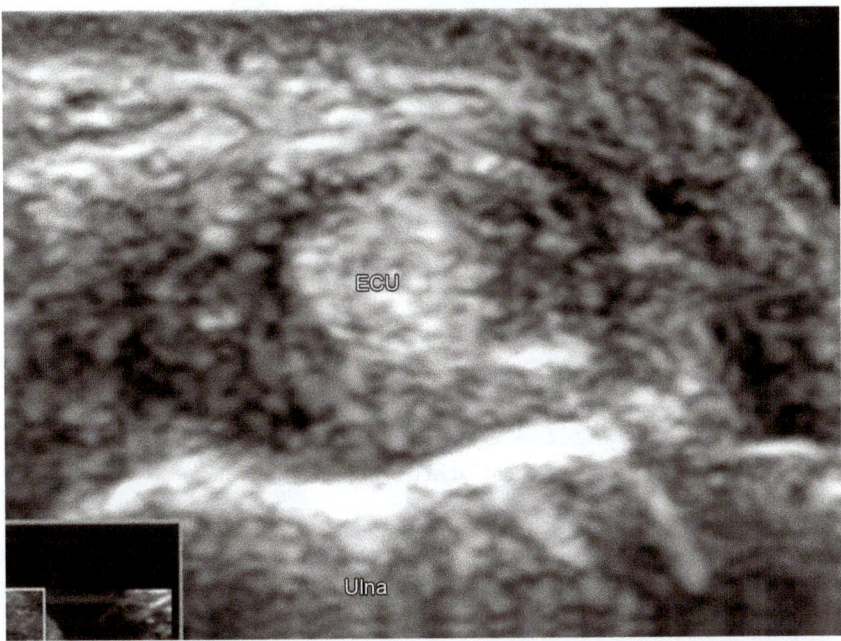

Fig. 3: Transverse image along the dorsal aspect of the wrist shows echogenic soft tissue within the extensor compartment VI tendon sheath. (ECU: extensor carpi ulnaris)

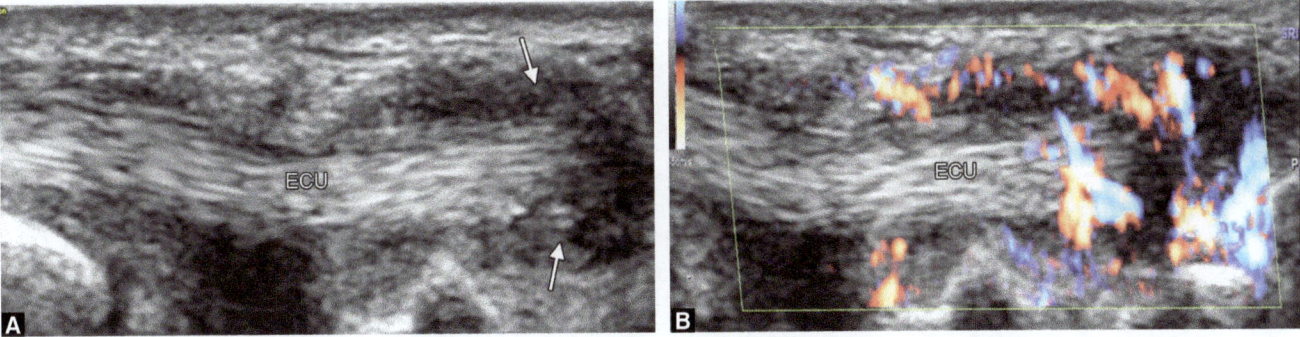

Figs. 4A and B: Long-axis images along the dorsal and ulnar aspect of the wrist show echogenic soft tissue within the extensor compartment VI tendon sheath. Power Doppler shows significant neovascularity within the thickened synovium. (ECU: extensor carpi ulnaris)

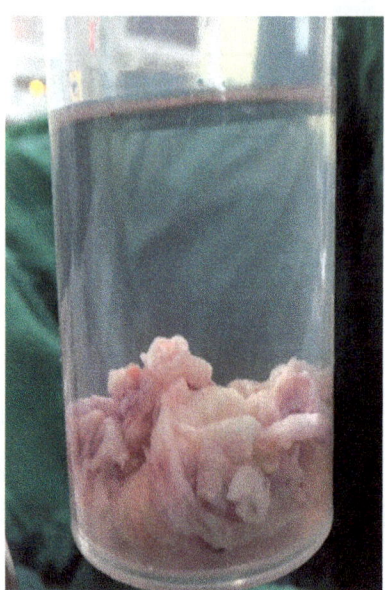

Fig. 5: Excised synovium.

Case 36

Epidermal Inclusion Cyst

CLINICAL HISTORY

A 46-year-old woman presented with painless firm nodule along the extensor aspect of the little finger (Fig. 1).

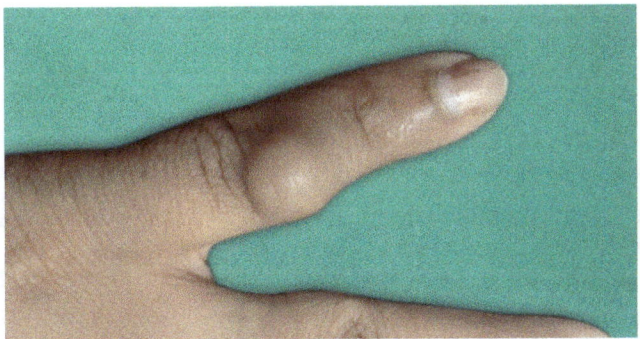

Fig. 1: Painless firm nodule along the dorsal aspect of finger.

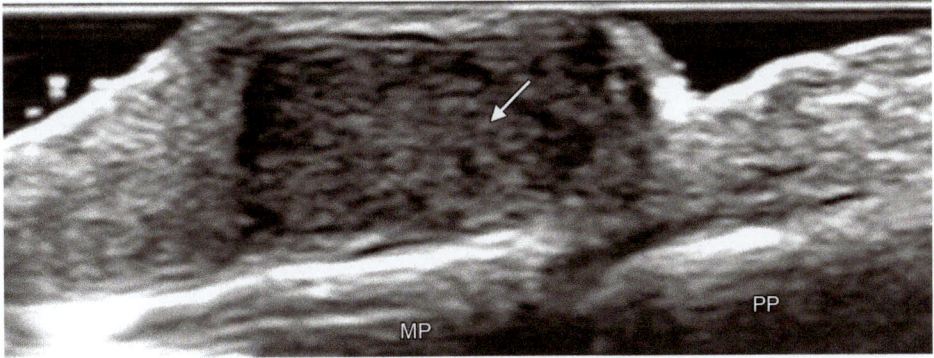

Fig. 2: Complex cyst (arrow) seen at the dorsal surface of the metacarpophalangeal joint. (MP: middle phalanx; PP: proximal phalanx)

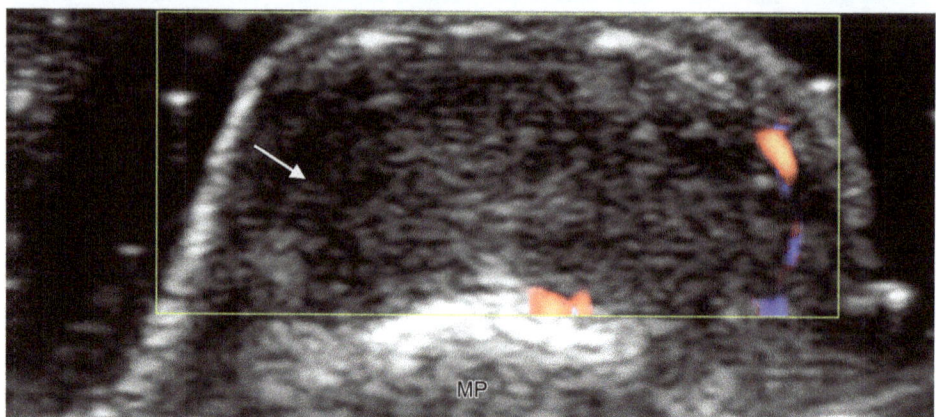

Fig. 3: Short-axis view with power Doppler does not show any significant intralesional vascularity. Arrow points to the inclusion cyst. (MP: middle phalanx)

◼ DIAGNOSIS

Epidermal inclusion cyst.

◼ DISCUSSION

- Epidermal inclusion cyst is the most common dermal cyst caused due to proliferation of squamous epithelium. The term sebaceous cyst for this lesion is a misnomer.
- These cysts are commonly occurs over the scalp, face, neck, trunk, and back.
- *Ultrasound (US) findings in epidermal inclusion cysts*:
    - Homogeneous and hypoechoic cystic lesions with low-level internal echoes.
    - Increased through transmission.
    - Internal linear echogenic reflections (Fig. 2).
    - Intralesional dark clefts may be seen in some cases.
    - Absence of intralesional vascularity on Doppler images (Fig. 3).

Case 37

Trigger Finger

CLINICAL HISTORY

A 52-year-old woman presented with stiffness in the right ring finger during extension. A snapping sensation was felt within the finger during extension.

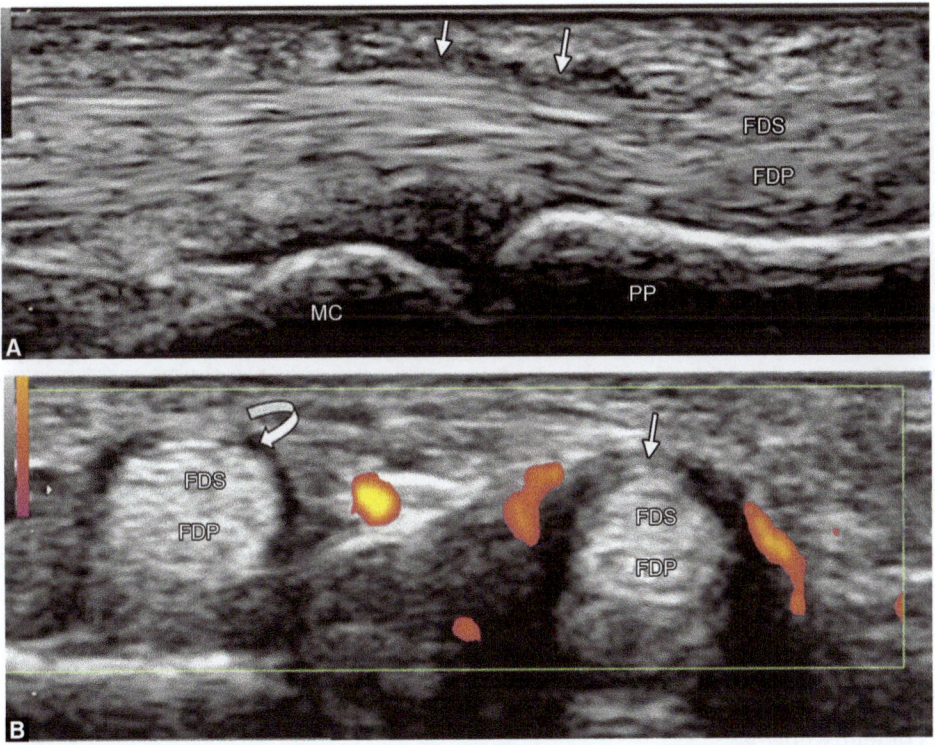

Figs. 1A and B: Long-axis (A) and transverse (B) images at the level of the metacarpophalangeal joint show diffuse thickening of the A1 pulley (arrows) along with increased vascularity on power Doppler (B). Comparison with the adjacent finger shows normal appearance of the A1 pulley (curved arrow). (FDP: flexor digitorum profundus; FDS: flexor digitorum superficialis; PP: proximal phalanx; MC: metacarpal head)

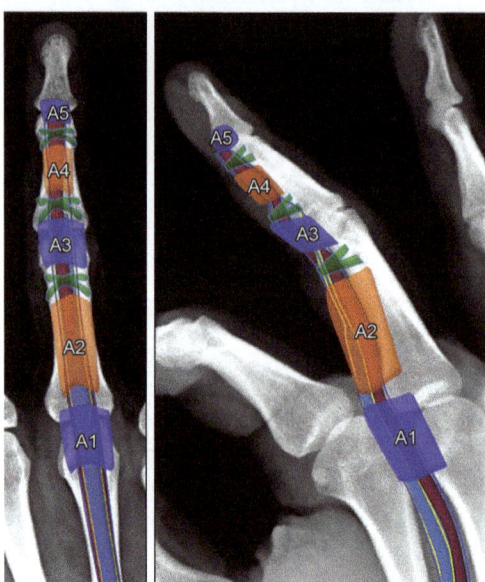

Fig. 2: Anatomy and location of pulleys along the finger—Annular pulleys (A1, A2, A3, A4, and A5), cruciate pulleys (green markers), flexor digitorum superficialis tendon (blue), and flexor digitorum profundus (dark red).

DIAGNOSIS

Trigger finger due to thickened A1 pulley.

DISCUSSION

- Anatomically, pulleys are characterized by localized thickening of the flexor tendon sheath along the volar aspect of the fingers. With the exception of the thumb, all the fingers have five annular and three cruciate pulleys (Fig. 2). The function of pulleys is to prevent bowstringing of the flexor tendons and keep them apposed to the phalanges and the joints during flexion.
- The A1 pulley is located at the metacarpophalangeal joint of all the fingers (including the thumb).
- Trigger finger is most commonly caused due to thickening of the A1 pulley.
- Chondroid metaplasia results in thickening of the pulleys (usually the A1 pulley), resulting in stenosing tenosynovitis.
- Trigger finger is usually associated with diabetes mellitus, hypothyroidism, amyloidosis, and connective tissue disorders.
- *Sonographic appearance of TFs*:
  - Thickened A1 pulley (thickness varies from 1.1 mm to 2.9 mm) (Fig. 1A).
  - Increased vascularity in the A1 pulley (Fig. 1B).
  - Tendinosis or tenosynovitis.
  - Cyst arising from the synovial sheath.
- Management of TF includes localized steroid injection or release of A1 pulley. These procedures may be done under ultrasound guidance.

FURTHER READING

1. Doyle JR. Anatomy of the finger flexor tendon sheath and pulley system. J Hand Surg Am. 1988;13:473-84.
2. Hauger O, Chung CB, Lektrakul N, et al. Pulley system in the fingers: normal anatomy and simulated lesions in cadavers at MR imaging, CT, and US with and without contrast material distention of the tendon sheath. Radiology. 2000;217:201-12.

Case 38

Trigger Thumb

CLINICAL HISTORY

A 48-year-old man with history of rheumatoid arthritis, presented with difficulty in extension of the right thumb, and intermittent pain along the volar aspect.

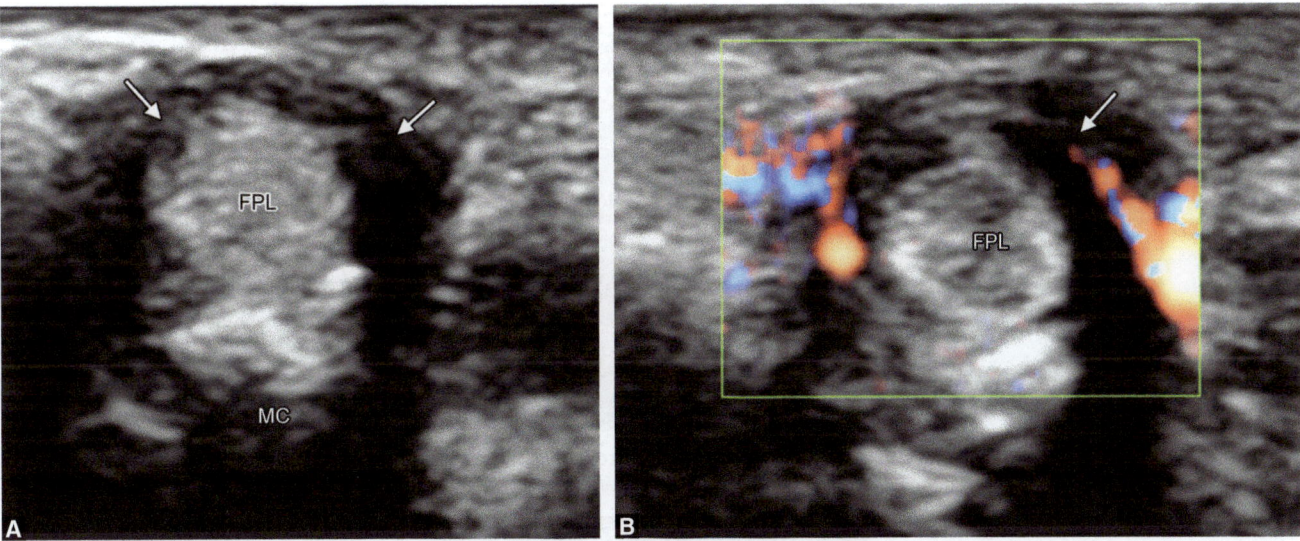

Figs. 1A and B: Transverse images at the level of the metacarpophalangeal joint show diffuse thickening (A) of the A1 pulley (arrows) along with neovascularity (B). (FPL: flexor pollicis longus; MC: metacarpal head)

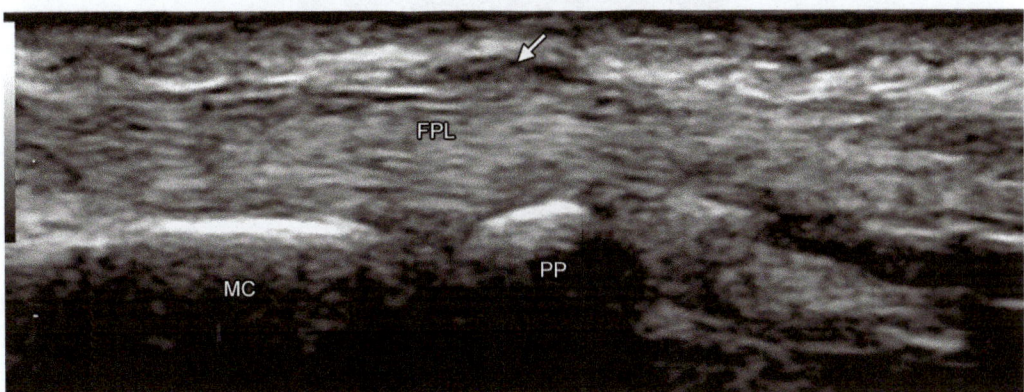

Fig. 2: Long-axis image showing thickened A1 pulley (arrow).
(FPL: flexor pollicis longus; PP: proximal phalanx; MC: metacarpal head)

DIAGNOSIS

Trigger thumb due to inflammation of A1 pulley.

Case 39

Crystal Deposition Disease

CLINICAL HISTORY

A 29-year-old man presented with an acute erythematous painful swelling along the right thenar eminence. There was no history of trauma.

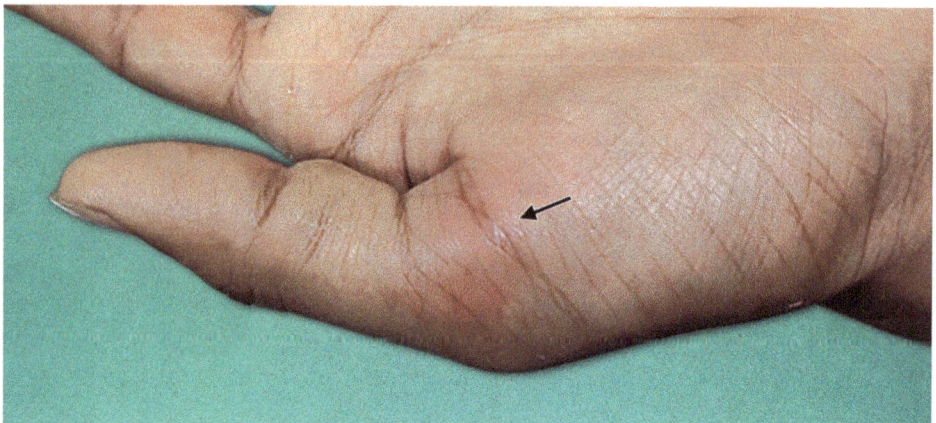

Fig. 1: Erythematous tender swelling (arrow) along the thenar eminence.

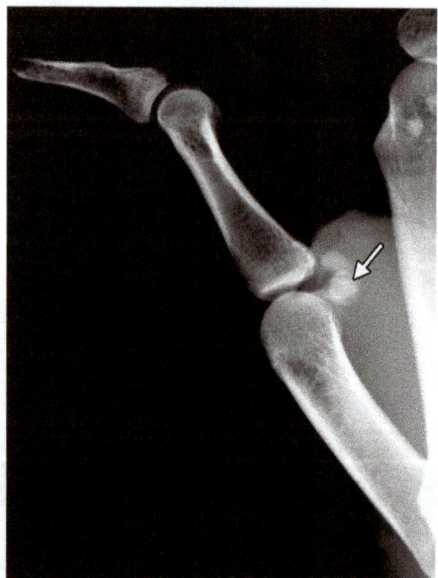

Fig. 2: Focal calcification along the volar aspect of the first metacarpophalangeal joint adjacent to the sesamoid bones.

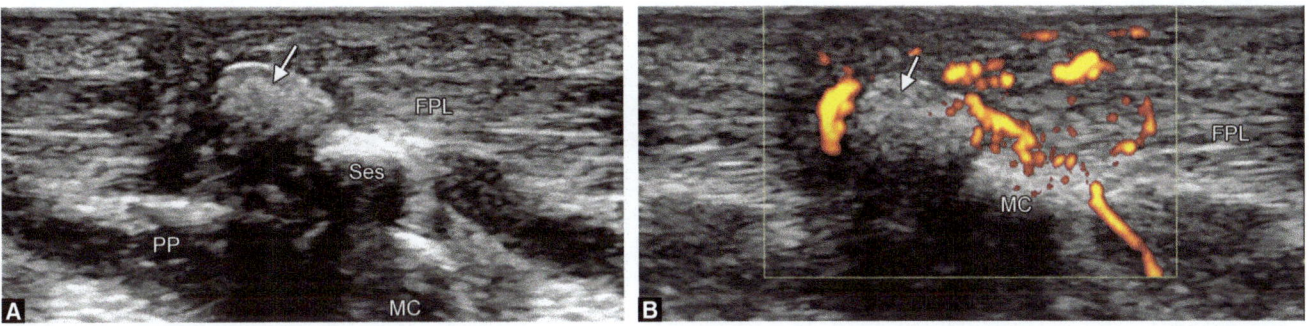

Figs. 3A and B: (A) Long-axis view shows periarticular calcium deposition (arrow) along the flexor pollicis longus (FPL) tendon. Ill-defined edema is seen in the periarticular planes; (B) Power Doppler shows marked neovascularity adjacent to the calcium (arrow). (MC: metacarpal head; PP: proximal phalanx; Ses: sesamoid)

DIAGNOSIS

Pericapsular crystal deposition disease.

DISCUSSION

- Hydroxyapatite crystal deposition is most commonly seen in the periarticular regions. Meanwhile, calcium pyrophosphate dihydrate (CPPD) typically involves the hyaline cartilage and the fibrocartilage.
- Hydroxyapatite crystal deposition is typically seen in bursae, tendons, and the periarticular soft tissues.
- On radiography, early HA crystal deposits appear as poorly defined amorphous calcific foci.
- On ultrasound (US), the periarticular deposits are seen as mildly echogenic nonshadowing foci.
- *Other findings on US*:
  - Periarticular edema.
  - Hyperemia on power Doppler images.
  - Reactive joint effusion.

Case 40

Ganglion Arising from the A2 Pulley

CLINICAL HISTORY

A 38-year-old woman presented with focal pain along the volar aspect of the finger since 2 months.

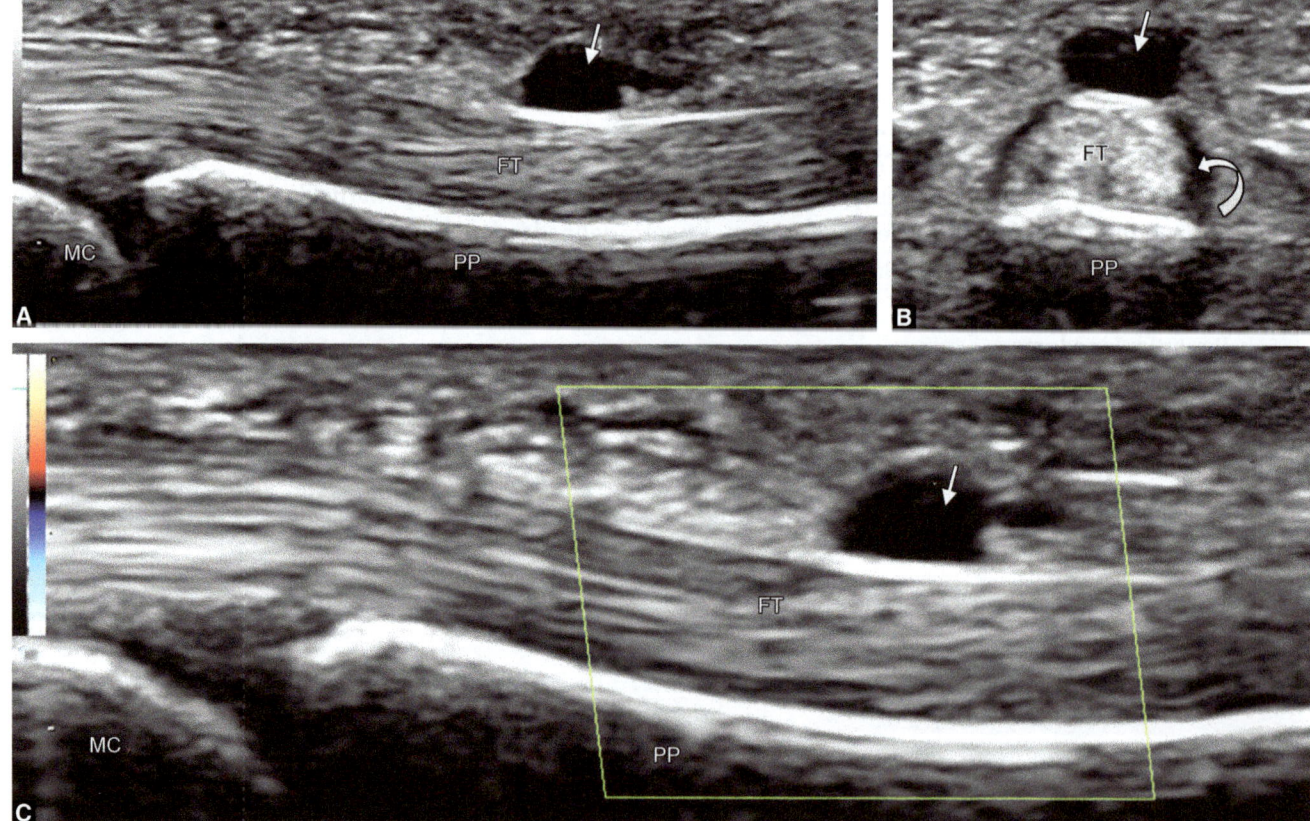

Figs. 1A to C: Long-axis (A and C) and transverse (B) images show a ganglion cyst (arrows) arising from the A2 pulley (curved arrow). (FT: flexor tendons; MC: metacarpal head; PP: proximal phalanx)

DIAGNOSIS

Ganglion arising from the A2 pulley.

Case 41

Nodular Thickening of the A2 Pulley in a Known Case of Rheumatoid Arthritis

CLINICAL HISTORY

A 47-year-old woman with history of rheumatoid arthritis presented with focal pain along the volar aspect of the left index finger since 8 months. The pain was aggravated during flexion and extension of the finger.

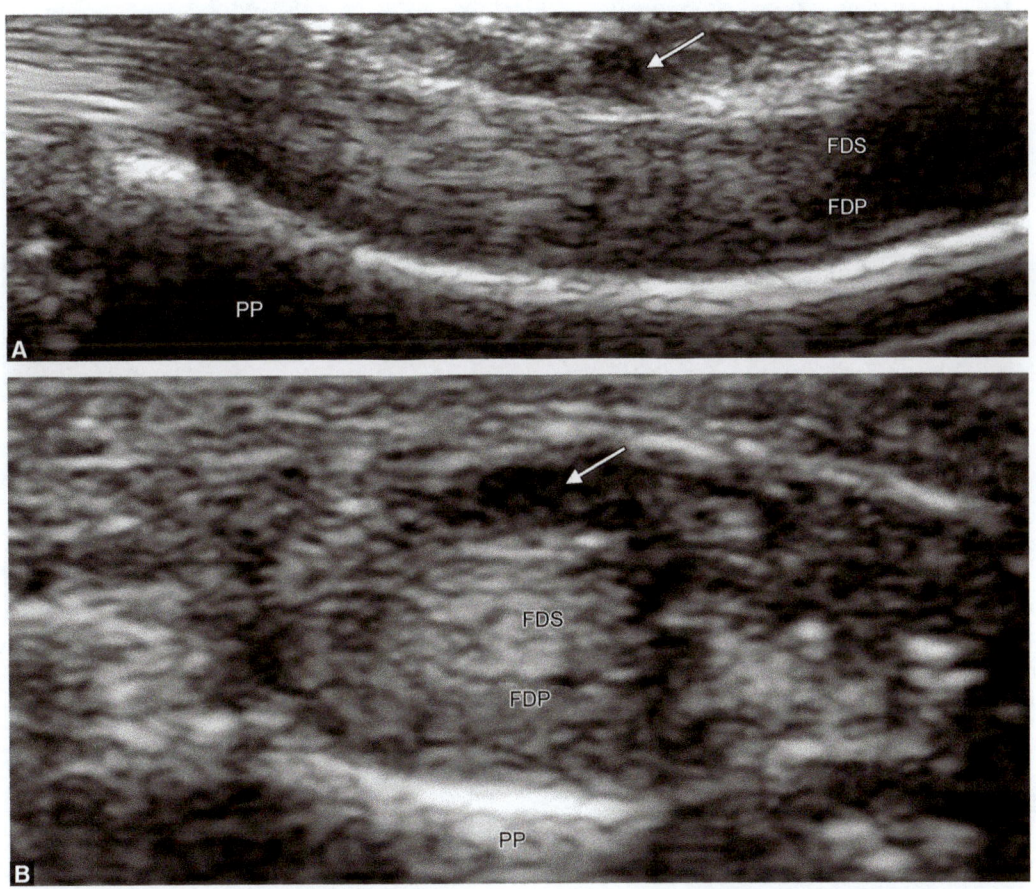

Figs. 1A and B: Long axis (A) and transverse (B) images show focal nodular thickening (arrows) of the A2 pulley. (FDS: flexor digitorum superficialis; FDP: flexor digitorum profundus; PP: proximal phalanx)

DIAGNOSIS

Nodular thickening of the A2 pulley.

CASE 42

Inflammatory Synovitis Involving the Metacarpophalangeal Joint

CLINICAL HISTORY

A 39-year-old woman with rheumatoid arthritis presented with stiffness of the left index finger since 2 months.

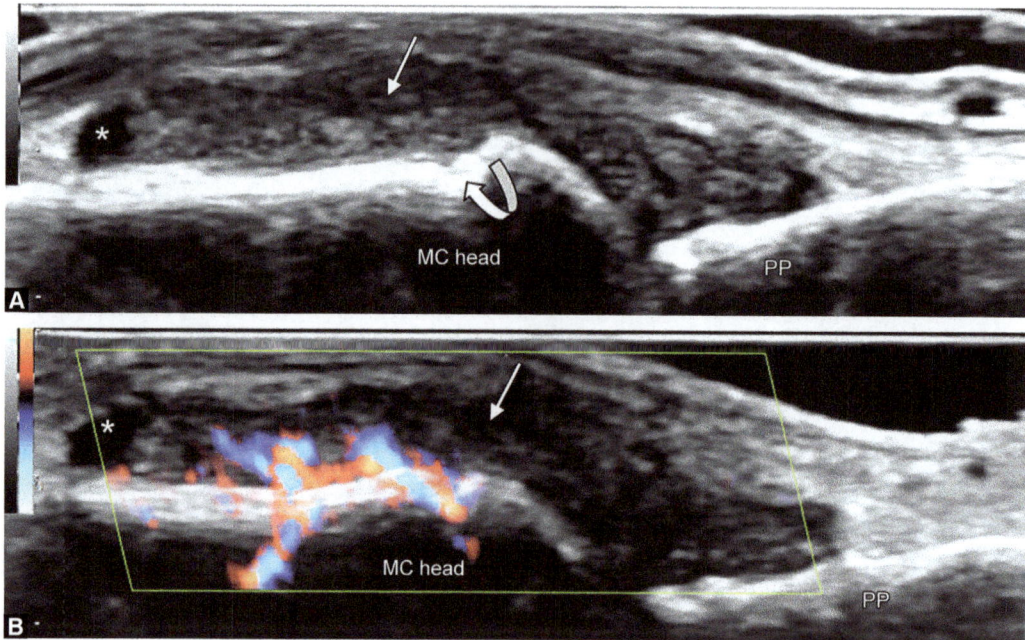

Figs. 1A and B: (A) Long-axis image of the dorsal recess of the metacarpophalangeal joint shows synovial hypertrophy (arrow), joint effusion (*), and large erosions (curved arrow) along the dorsal cortex of the metacarpal (MC) head; (B) Power Doppler shows grade 2 vascularity within the thickened synovium. (PP: proximal phalanx)

DIAGNOSIS

Inflammatory arthropathy (rheumatoid arthritis) involving the metacarpophalangeal joint of the index finger.

DISCUSSION

- In rheumatology, musculoskeletal ultrasound (US) is widely used in the detection and management of inflammatory arthritis.[1]

- Proliferative synovitis (rheumatoid pannus) is the earliest pathologic abnormality in inflammatory arthritis, secondarily responsible for bone and cartilage damage.
- *Pathological findings on US in inflammatory arthropathies*:
  - Synovial effusion (Figs. 1A and B)
  - Synovial hypertrophy
  - Tenosynovitis
  - Tendinosis
  - Erosions (Figs. 1,2 and 4).
- The Outcome Measures in Rheumatoid Arthritis Clinical Trial (OMERACT) scoring system is used for US synovial changes.
- *The OMERACT definitions of various pathological findings on US*:
  - *Synovial fluid* is an abnormal hypoechoic or anechoic intra-articular material that is displaceable and compressible and does not exhibit Doppler signal.[2]
  - *Synovial hypertrophy* appears as a hypoechoic tissue that is not displaceable and poorly compressible and may exhibit Doppler signal.[1]
  - *Erosions* are defined as intra-articular discontinuities of the bone surface visible in two perpendicular planes.[2]
  - *Tenosynovitis* is a hypo/anechoic tissue with/without fluid within the tendon sheath, which is seen in two perpendicular planes and may exhibit a Doppler signal (Figs. 3 and 4).[2]
- Both clinical and subclinical US detected synovitis (neovascularity on power Doppler) have more predictive value (compared to the radiological erosions, flares) than clinical assessment.

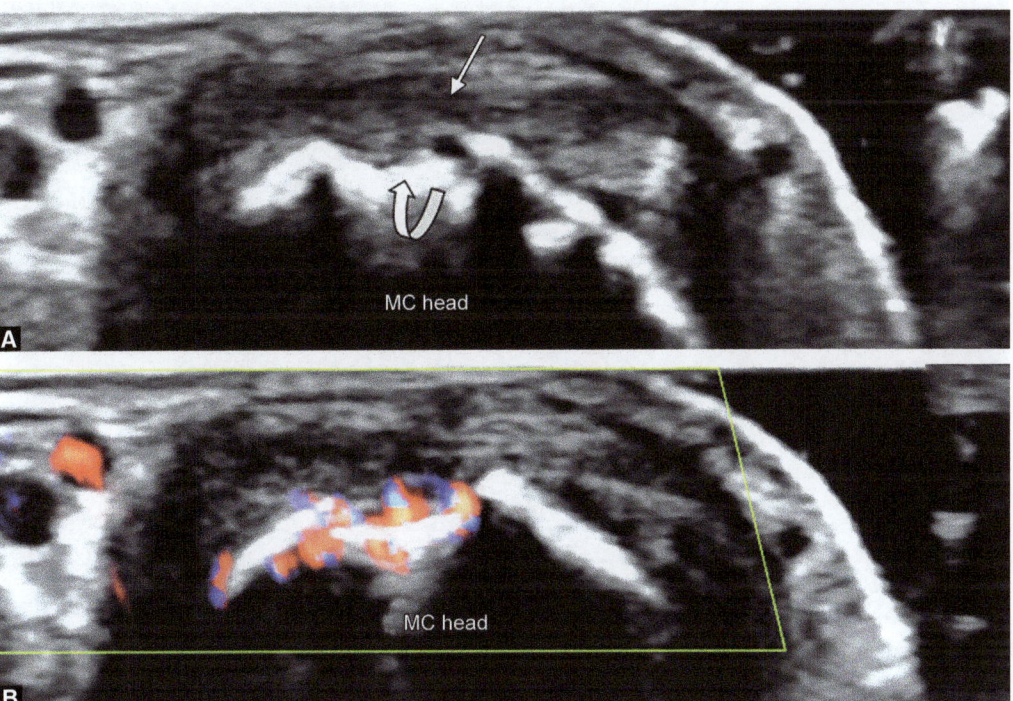

Figs. 2A and B: (A) Transverse image of the dorsal recess of the metacarpophalangeal joint shows synovial hypertrophy (arrow), and large erosions (curved arrow) along the dorsal cortex of the metacarpal (MC) head; (B) Power Doppler shows vascularity within the thickened synovium.

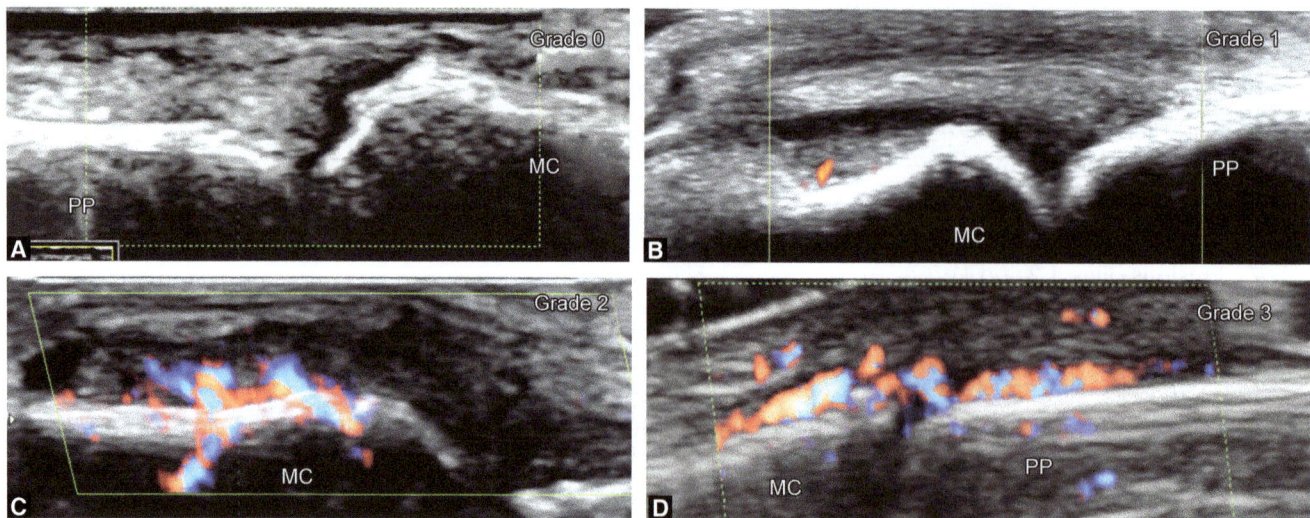

Figs. 3A to D: (A) *Grade 0:* No flow in the synovium; (B) *Grade 1:* Up to three single spot signals or up to two confluent spots or one confluent spot + up to two single spots; (C) *Grade 2:* Vessel signals in less than half of the area of the synovium (<50%); and (D) *Grade 3:* Vessel signals in more than half of the area of the synovium (>50%). (MC: metacarpal head; PP: proximal phalanx)

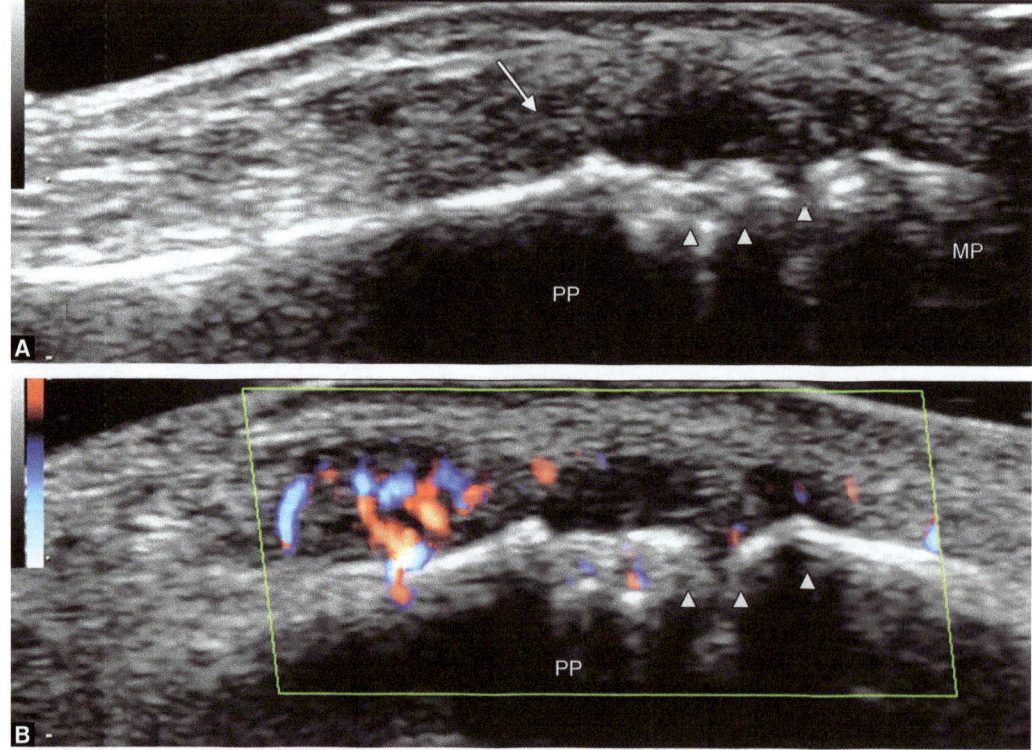

Figs. 4A and B: (A) Long-axis image of the dorsal recess of the interphalangeal joint shows synovial hypertrophy (arrow) and large erosions (arrowheads) along the dorsal cortex of the proximal phalanx (PP); (B) Power Doppler shows grade 2 vascularity within the thickened synovium. (MP: middle phalanx)

- *Criteria for US monitoring of therapy:*
  - Reduction in thickness of pannus
  - Change in neovascularity
  - Erosions.
- Ultrasound is more sensitive than radiography in detection of bone erosions in accessible joints (second and fifth metacarpophalangeal joints and proximal interphalangeal joint).

REFERENCES

1. Kane D, Grassi W, Sturrock R, et al. Musculoskeletal ultrasound—a state of the art review in rheumatology. Part 2: Clinical indications for musculoskeletal ultrasound in rheumatology. Rheumatology (Oxford). 2004;43:829-38.
2. Wakefield RJ, Balint PV, Szudlarek M, et al. Musculoskeletal ultrasound including definitions for ultrasonographic pathology. J Rheumatol. 2005;32:2485-7.

Case 43

Tenosynovitis with Tendinosis of the Flexor Tendons of the Finger due to a Retained Foreign Body

■ CLINICAL HISTORY

A 26-year-old woman presented with painful swelling of the left middle finger. There is a history of glass injury 3 years ago.

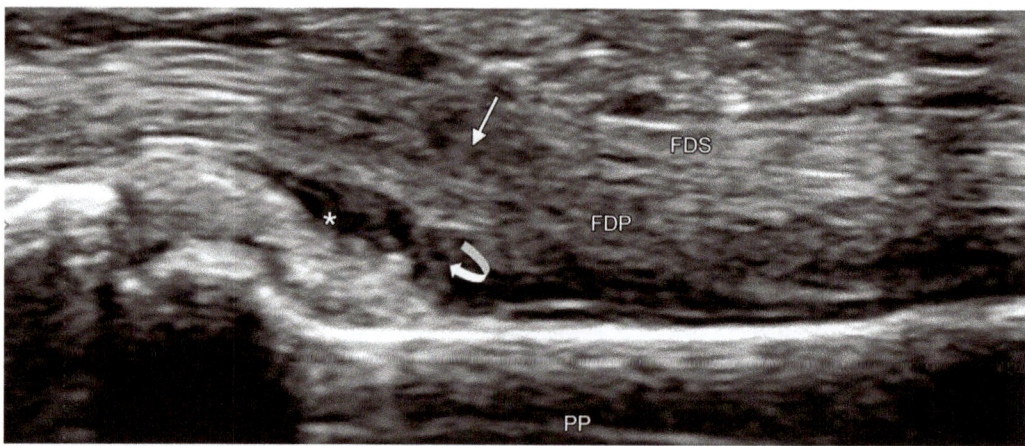

Fig. 1: Long-axis image along the volar aspect of the finger shows effusion (*) and synovial hypertrophy (curved arrow) within flexor tendon sheath. The flexor digitorum superficialis (FDS) and flexor digitorum profundus (FDP) tendons appear thickened (arrow) and loss of echogenic pattern. (PP: proximal phalanx)

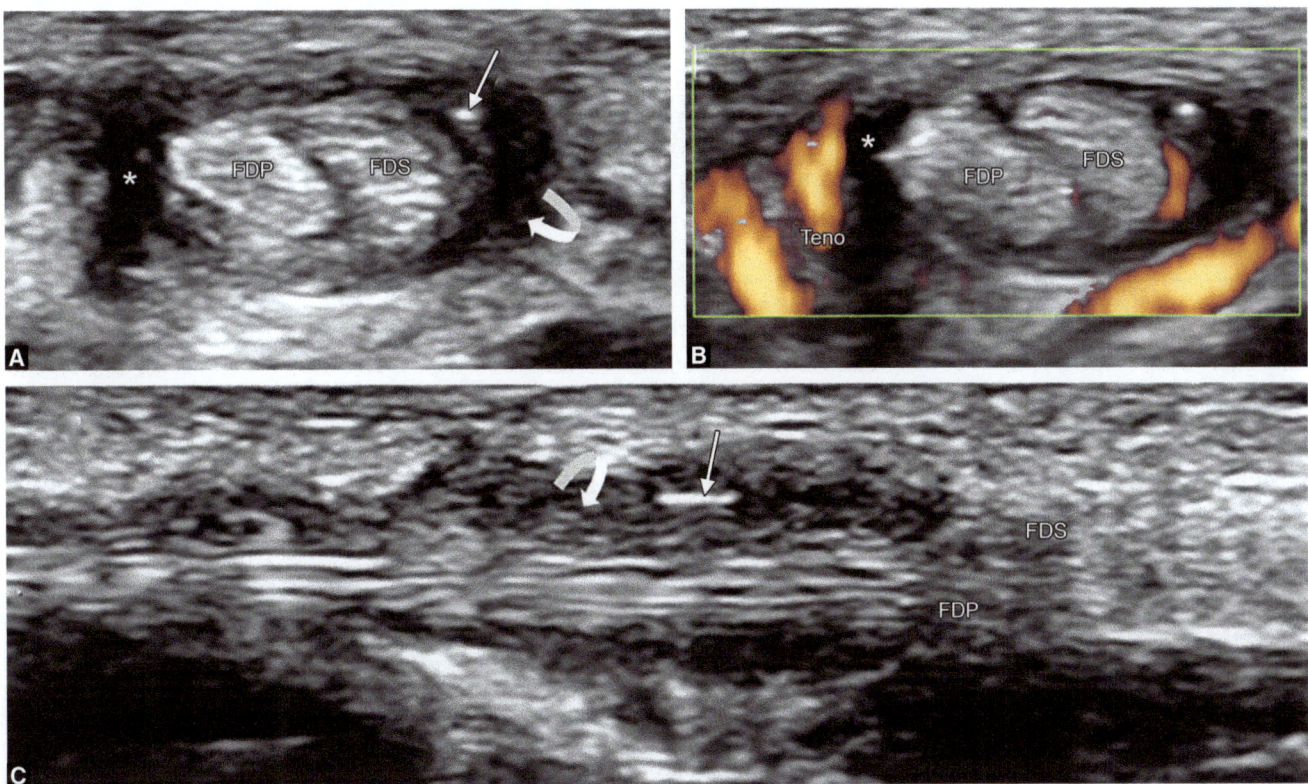

Figs. 2A to C: Transverse (A and B) and long-axis (C) images along the volar aspect of the finger show effusion (*) and synovial hypertrophy (curved arrows) within flexor tendon sheath. An echogenic linear foreign body (arrows) is seen within the thickened synovium. (FDS: flexor digitorum superficialis; FDP: flexor digitorum profundus; Teno: tenosynovitis)

■ DIAGNOSIS

Tenosynovitis of the flexor tendons of the middle finger along with tendinosis due to a retained foreign body.

Case 44

Traumatic Full-thickness Tear of Flexor Digitorum Profundus Tendon

■ CLINICAL HISTORY

A 28-year-old man presented with a penetrating injury along the flexor aspect of the index finger.

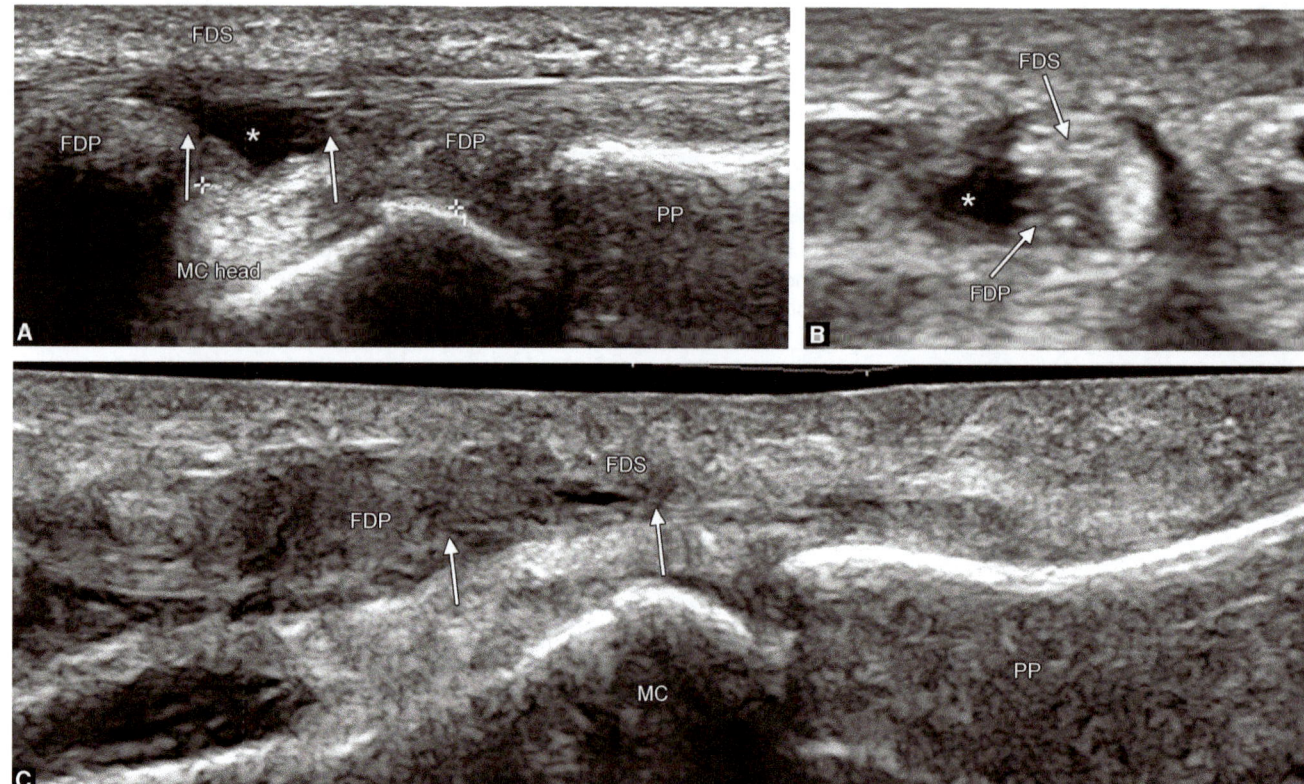

Figs. 1A to C: Long-axis (A and C) and transverse (B) images along the volar aspect of the finger show a full-thickness tear (*) of the flexor digitorum profundus (FDP) tendon. The defect (*) between the margins (arrows) of the torn FDP tendon is filled with fluid. The flexor digitorum superficialis (FDS) tendon appears intact. (MC: metacarpal head; PP: proximal phalanx)

■ DIAGNOSIS

Full-thickness tear of the flexor digitorum profundus tendon with proximal retraction of the torn tendon.

Case 45

Traumatic Full-thickness Tear of Extensor Pollicis Longus Tendon

CLINICAL HISTORY

A 50-year-old woman presented with a knife injury along the dorsal aspect of the thumb.

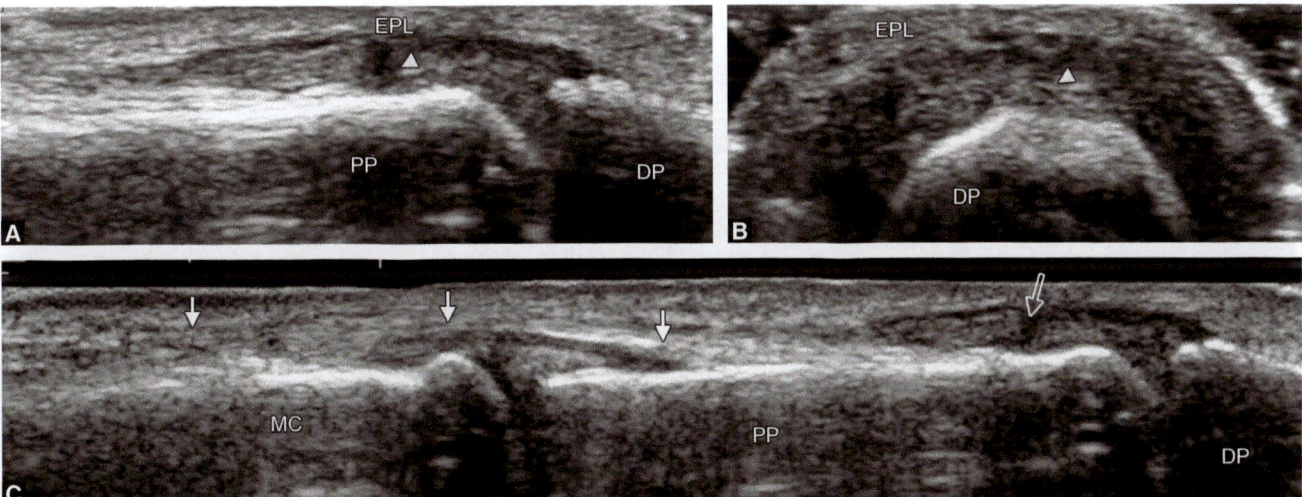

Figs. 1A to C: Long-axis images (A and C) and transverse image (B) along the dorsal aspect of the thumb show a full-thickness tear (arrowheads) of the extensor pollicis longus (EPL) tendon. (DP: distal phalanx; MC: metacarpal head; PP: proximal phalanx)

DIAGNOSIS

Full-thickness tear of the extensor pollicis longus tendon.

CASE 46

Giant-cell Tumor of Flexor-tendon Sheath of a Finger

■ CLINICAL HISTORY

A 29-year-old male presented with progressively increasing swelling along the volar aspect of the middle finger since 1 year.

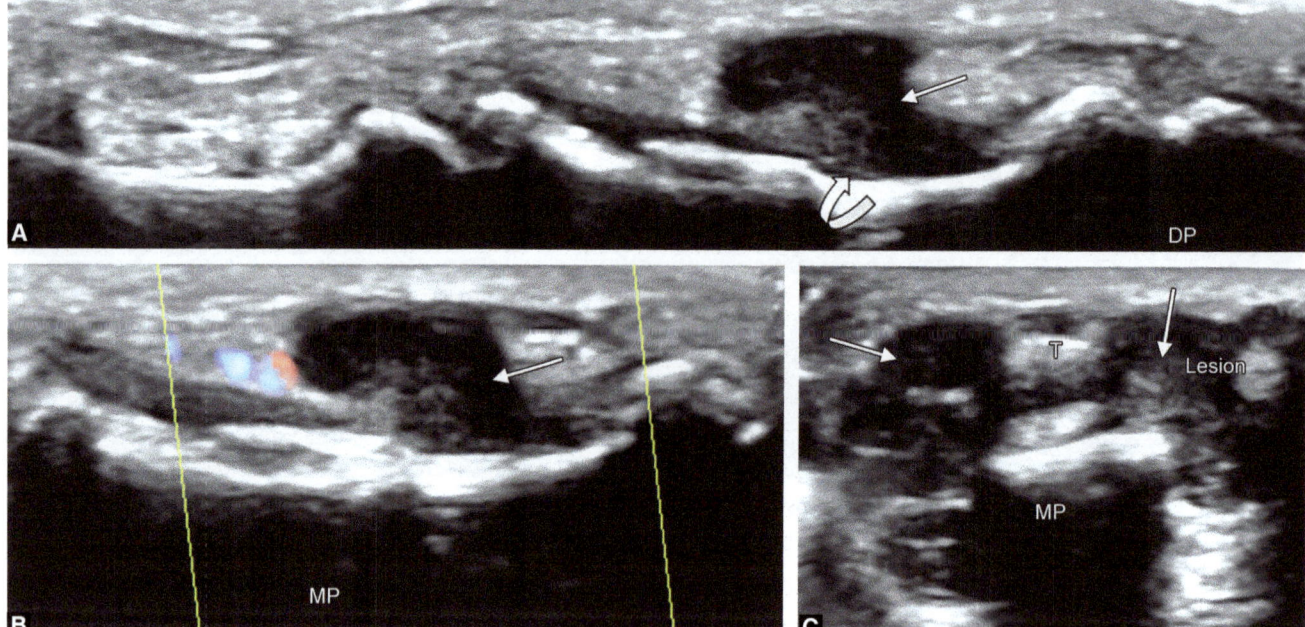

Figs. 1A to C: Hypoechoic soft tissue (straight arrows) seen encasing the flexor tendons (T) of the finger. The lesion is seen to cause cortical scalloping (curved arrow) of the underlying middle phalanx. Power Doppler does not show any significant intralesional vascularity. (DP: distal phalanx; MP: middle phalanx)

■ DIAGNOSIS

Giant-cell tumor (GCT) of the tendon sheath.

■ DISCUSSION

- Giant-cell tumor consists of multinucleated giant cells and hemosiderin aggregates. The locally aggressive lesion typically involves the synovium of the tendon sheath.
- *Ultrasound (US) findings*:
  - Well-defined hypoechoic mass encircling the tendon.
  - Intralesional vascularity (on power Doppler) is seen in most of the lesions.
  - Cortical scalloping of the adjacent bone may be seen.

Case 47

Giant-cell Tumor of Extensor Tendon of Finger

■ CLINICAL HISTORY

A 40-year-old female presented with dorsal aspect of the little finger since 1 year.

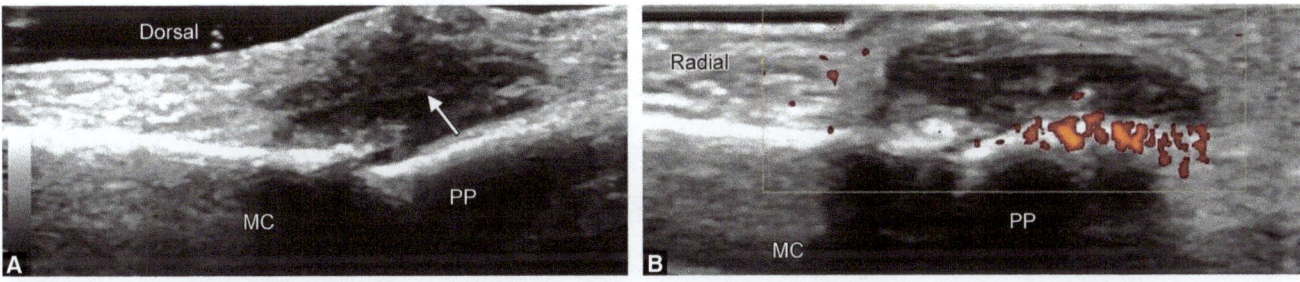

Figs. 1A and B: (A) Hypoechoic soft tissue (arrow) seen at the dorsal surface of the metacarpophalangeal joint along the radial aspect; and (B) Power Doppler shows intralesional vascularity. (MC: metacarpal head; PP: proximal phalanx)

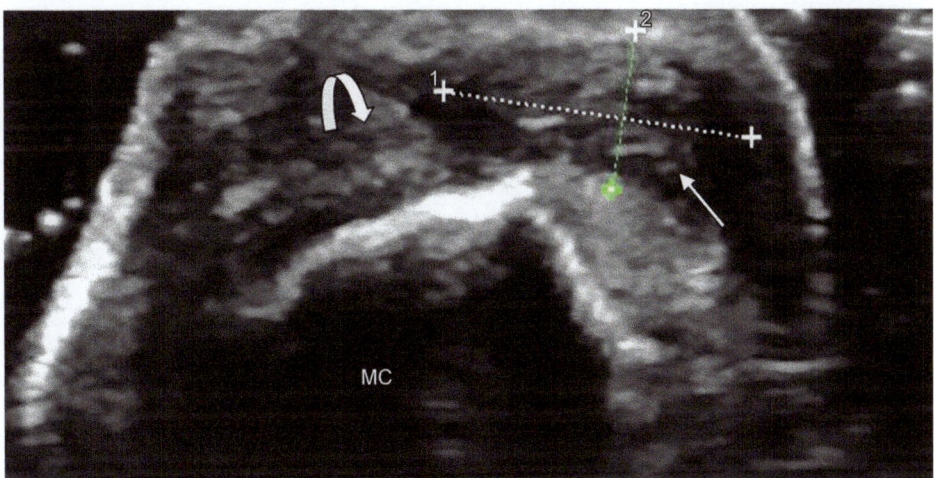

Fig. 2: Hypoechoic soft tissue (arrow) seen along the dorsal aspect of the metacarpophalangeal joint in close relation to the extensor tendon (curved arrow). (MC: metacarpal head)

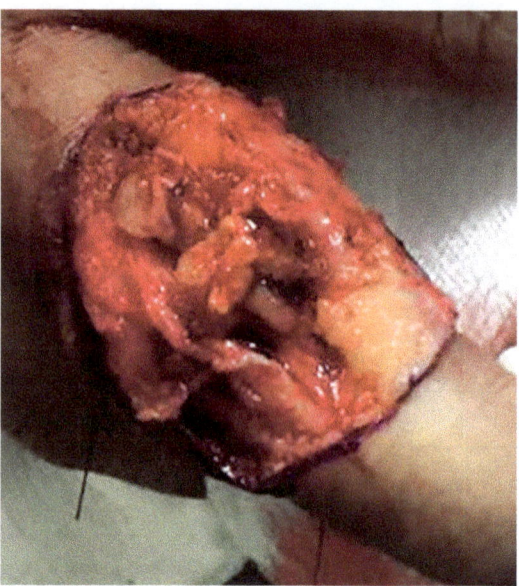

Fig. 3: Intraoperative image.

◼ DIAGNOSIS

Giant-cell tumor along the extensor tendon.

Case 48

Subungual Glomus Tumor

■ CLINICAL HISTORY

A 32-year-old woman presented with sharp pain along the tip of the right ring finger since 6 months. The pain was aggravated by local pressure and cold temperature. Clinical examination showed a bluish-red lesion below the nail bed.

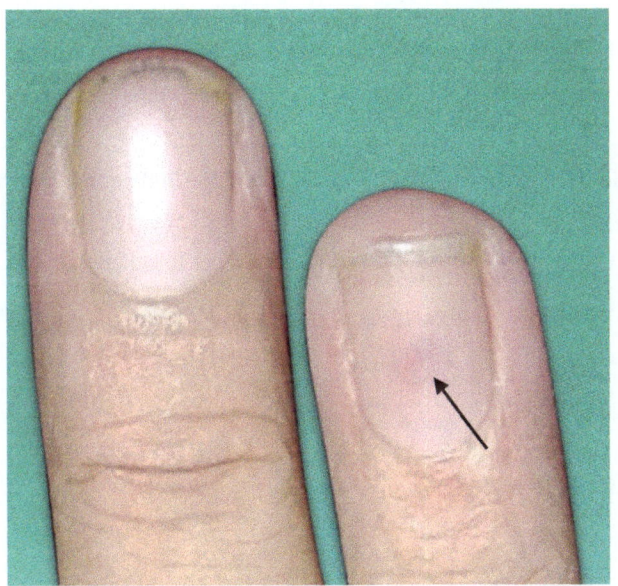

Fig. 1: Bluish-red colored tender lesion below the nail bed.

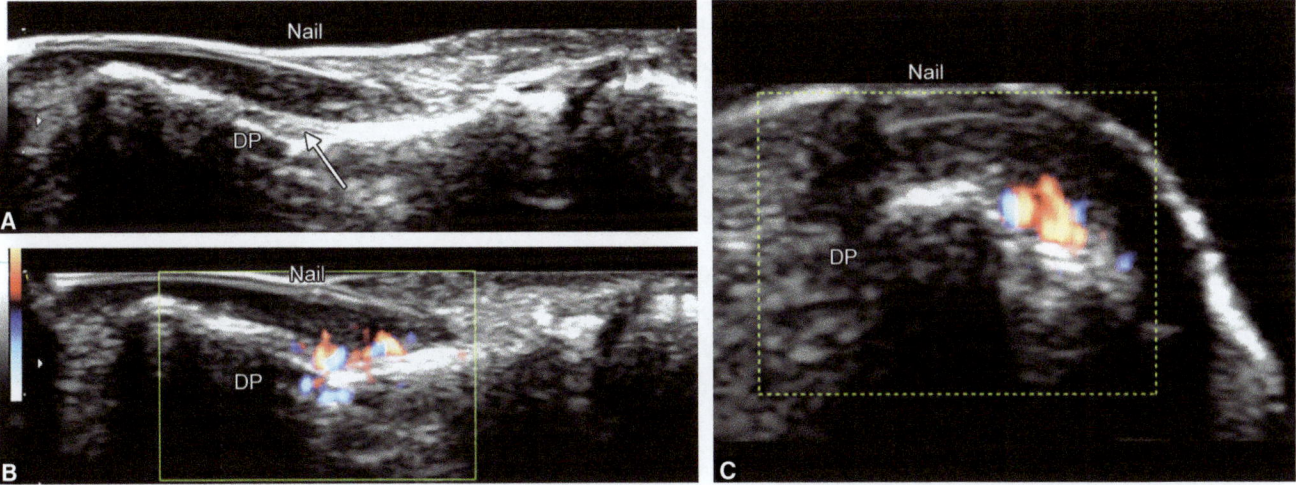

Figs. 2A to C: (A) Long-axis image shows an isoechoic lesion along the nail bed causing scalloping of the dorsal cortex (arrow) of the terminal phalanx; and (B and C) Power Doppler images show intense vascularity within the lesion. (DP: distal phalanx)

DIAGNOSIS

Subungual glomus tumor of the ring finger.

DISCUSSION

- Glomus tumor is a hamartoma arising from the neuromyoarterial glomus body.[1] It is a rare tumor.
- Glomus bodies consist of an afferent arteriole, a tortuous arteriovenous anastomosis, system of collecting veins, and neurovascular reticulum that regulates blood flow through the anastomosis.[1]
- Clinical presentation includes:
  - Severe pain in the affected finger.
  - Pinpoint tenderness.
  - Intense pain on exposure to cold temperature.
  - Bluish discoloration along the nail or fingertips.
- *Role of ultrasound (US) in evaluation of glomus tumors*:
  - Ultrasound allows localization of the glomus tumors. Ultrasound detect tumors as small as 3 mm.
  - Glomus tumors are seen as well-defined hypoechoic or isoechoic solid lesions in the subungual space.
  - Intense intralesional vascularity on power Doppler is a very specific finding for glomus tumors.
  - Cortical erosions or scalloping may be seen due to the mass effect by the tumor.

REFERENCE

1. Horcajadas AB, Lafuente JL, de la Cruz Burgos R, et al. Ultrasound and MR findings in tumor and tumor-like lesions of the fingers. Eur Radiol. 2003;13:672-85.

Case 49

Glomus Tumor

CLINICAL HISTORY

A 28-year-old woman presented with sharp pain along the nail bed of the left thumb. The pain was aggravated on exposure to cold water.

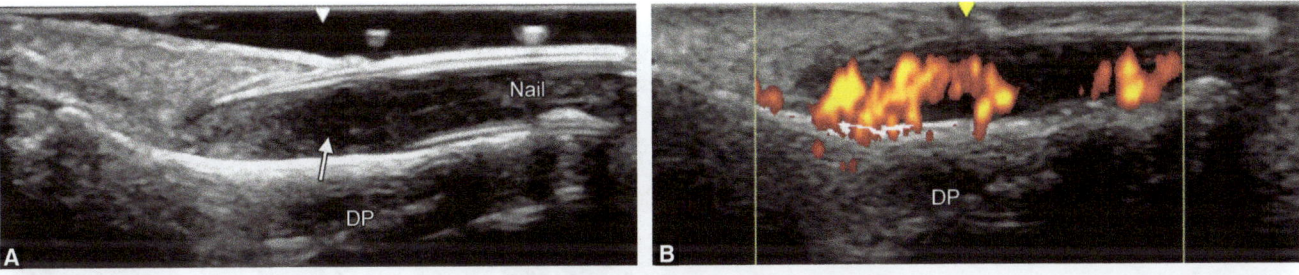

Figs. 1A and B: (A) Long-axis image shows an iso to hypoechoic lesion along the nail bed (arrow); and (B) Power Doppler image shows intense vascularity within the lesion. (DP: distal phalanx)

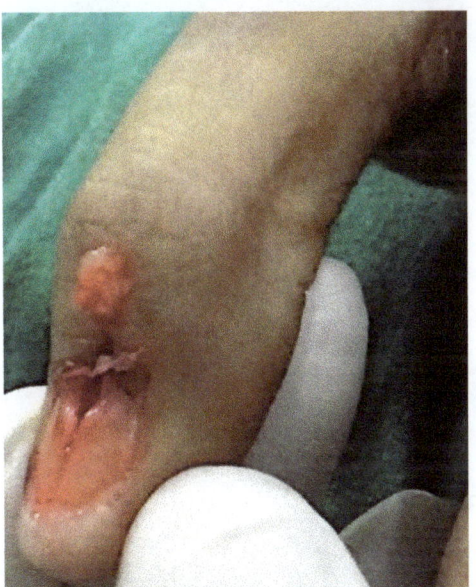

Fig. 2: Intraoperative image shows the excised glomus tumor.

DIAGNOSIS

Subungual glomus tumor of the thumb.

CASE 50

Avulsion Injury of Ulnar Collateral Ligament Injury of Thumb

■ CLINICAL HISTORY

A 46-year-old man presented with a painful erythematous swelling over the thenar eminence following a bike accident.

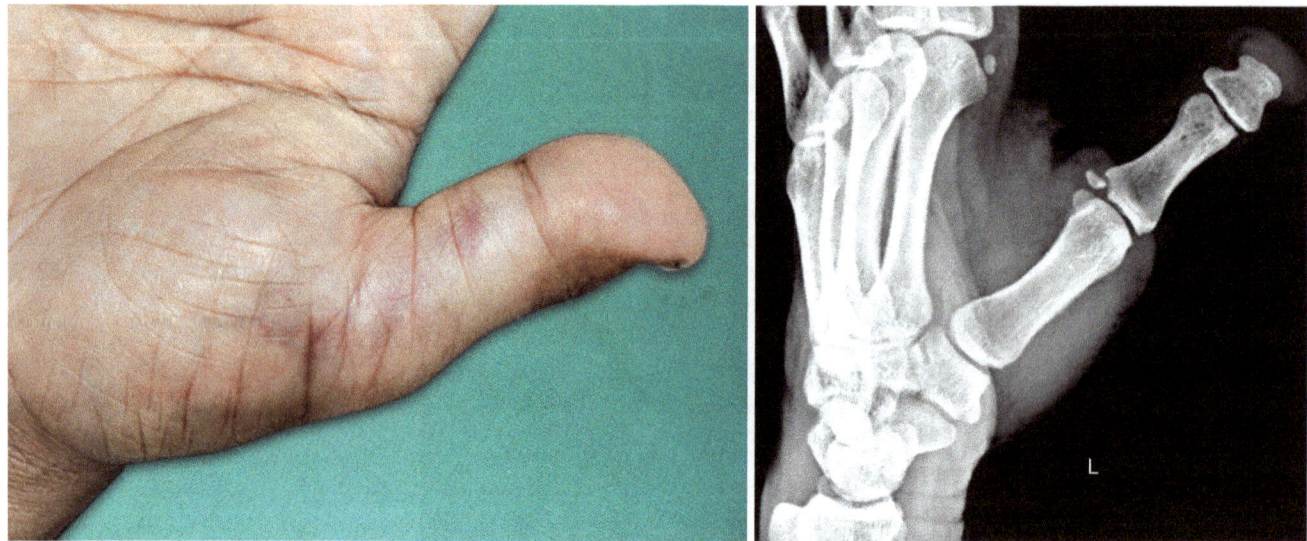

Fig. 1: Painful swelling along the thenar eminence with ecchymosis. The radiograph of the thumb shows a mildly displaced fracture along the base of the proximal phalanx.

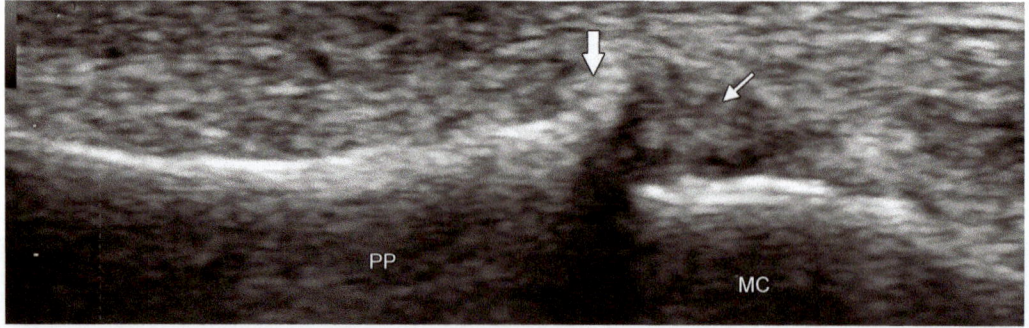

Fig. 2: Long-axis image along the ulnar aspect of the metacarpophalangeal joint shows a thickened ulnar collateral ligament (arrow). An osseous fragment is seen attached to the ulnar collateral ligament (solid arrow). (MC: metacarpal head; PP: proximal phalanx)

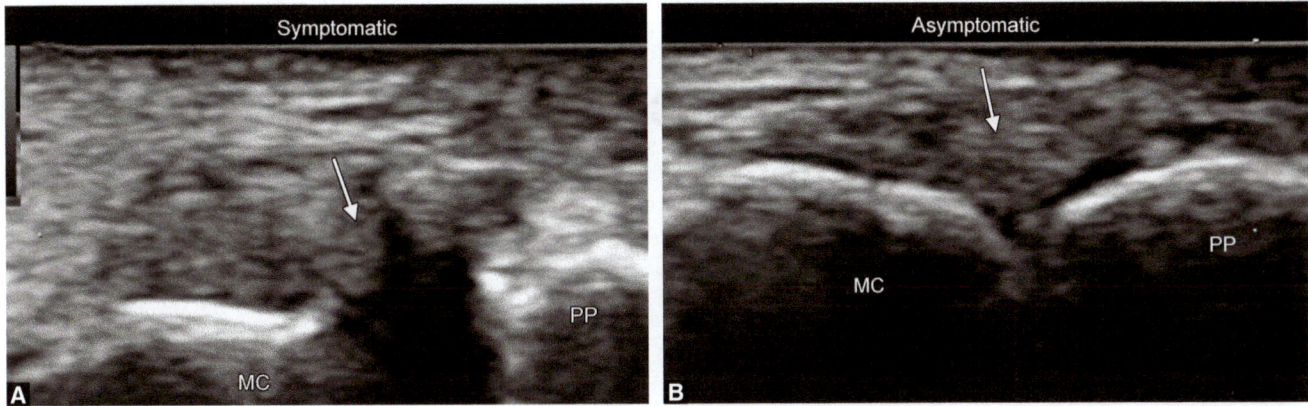

Figs. 3A and B: Comparison of long-axis view with the asymptomatic side shows normal appearance of the ulnar collateral ligament (arrows). (MC: metacarpal head; PP: proximal phalanx)

DIAGNOSIS

Skier's thumb (avulsion injury of the ulnar collateral ligament at the metacarpophalangeal joint).

CASE 51

Acute Partial-thickness Tear of the Adductor Muscles

CLINICAL HISTORY

A 67-year-old man presented with a painful erythematous swelling along the medial aspect of the left thigh extending proximally till the groin.

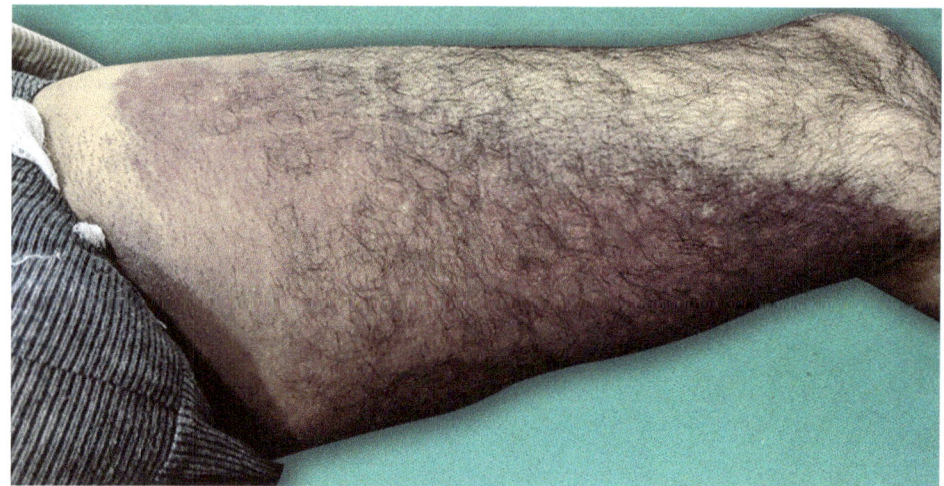

Fig. 1: Ill-defined swelling seen along the medial aspect of the thigh with ecchymosis.

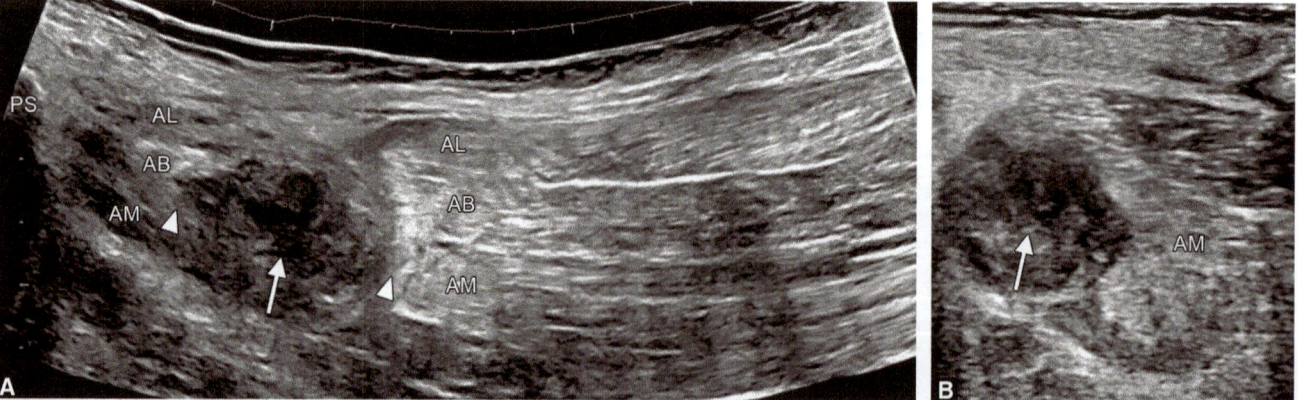

Figs. 2A and B: (A) Long-axis image shows a partial-thickness tear (arrow) of the adductor group of muscles. The tear predominantly involves the adductor magnus (AM) and adductor brevis (AB) muscle bellies. The torn edges (arrowheads) appear irregular; and (B) The defect caused due to the tear, is occupied by hematoma (arrow). (PS: pubic symphysis; AL: adductor longus)

DIAGNOSIS

Partial-thickness acute tear of the adductor muscles with a hematoma (Figs. 1 and 2).

ADDITIONAL CASE

CHRONIC PARTIAL THICKNESS TEAR AT THE COMMON ADDUCTOR ORIGIN

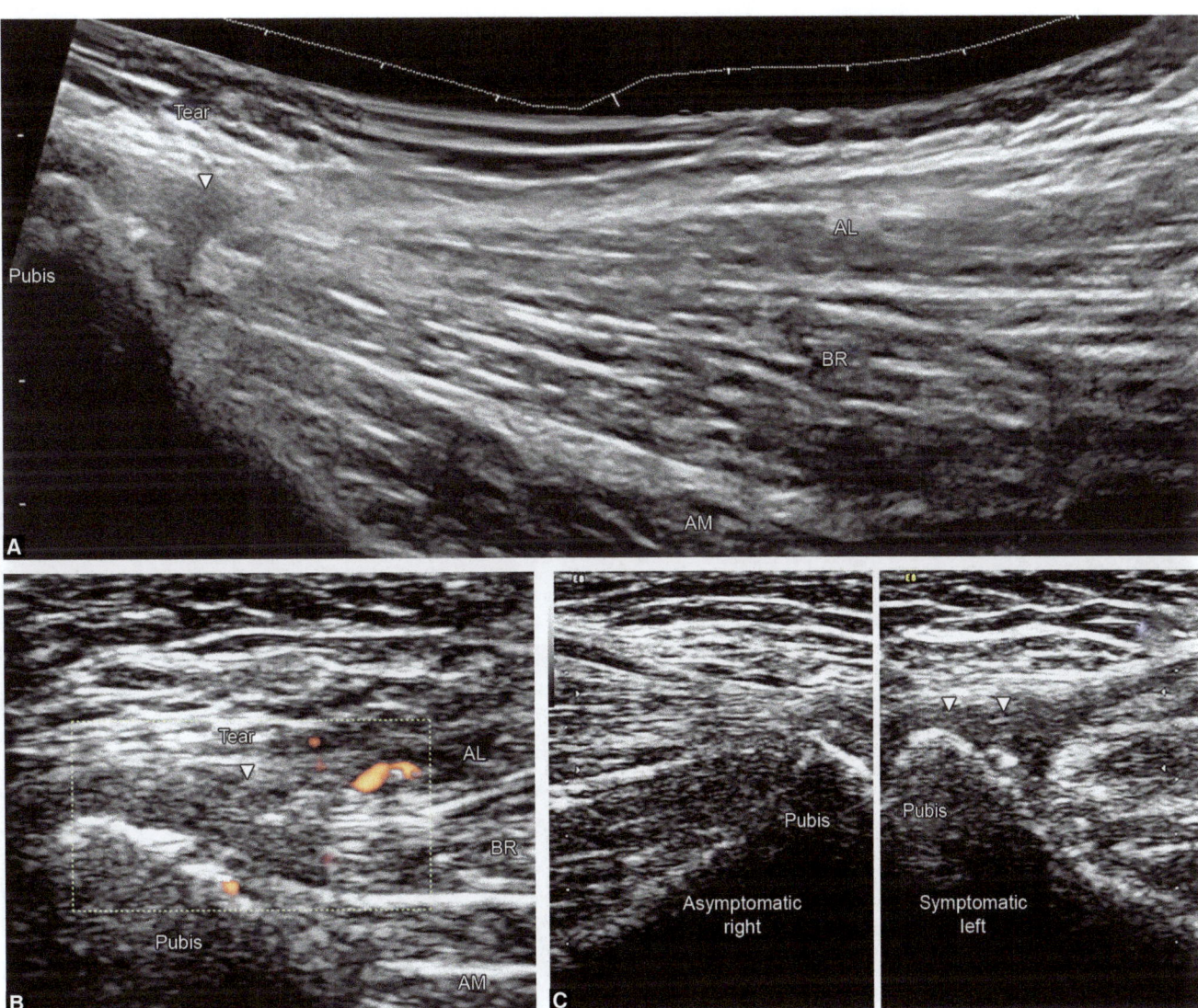

Figs. 3A to C: (A) Long-axis image shows a partial-thickness tear (arrowhead) at the adductor origin. The tear involves the adductor magnus (AM) and adductor longus (AL) muscles; (B) The torn edges show increased vascularity on power Doppler images; and (C) The tear appears more obvious (arrowheads) when comparison is made with the asymptomatic side. (BR: Adductor Brevis)

Case 52

Greater Trochanteric Bursitis

CLINICAL HISTORY

A 46-year-old man presented with pain along the lateral aspect of the right hip. There was no history of trauma.

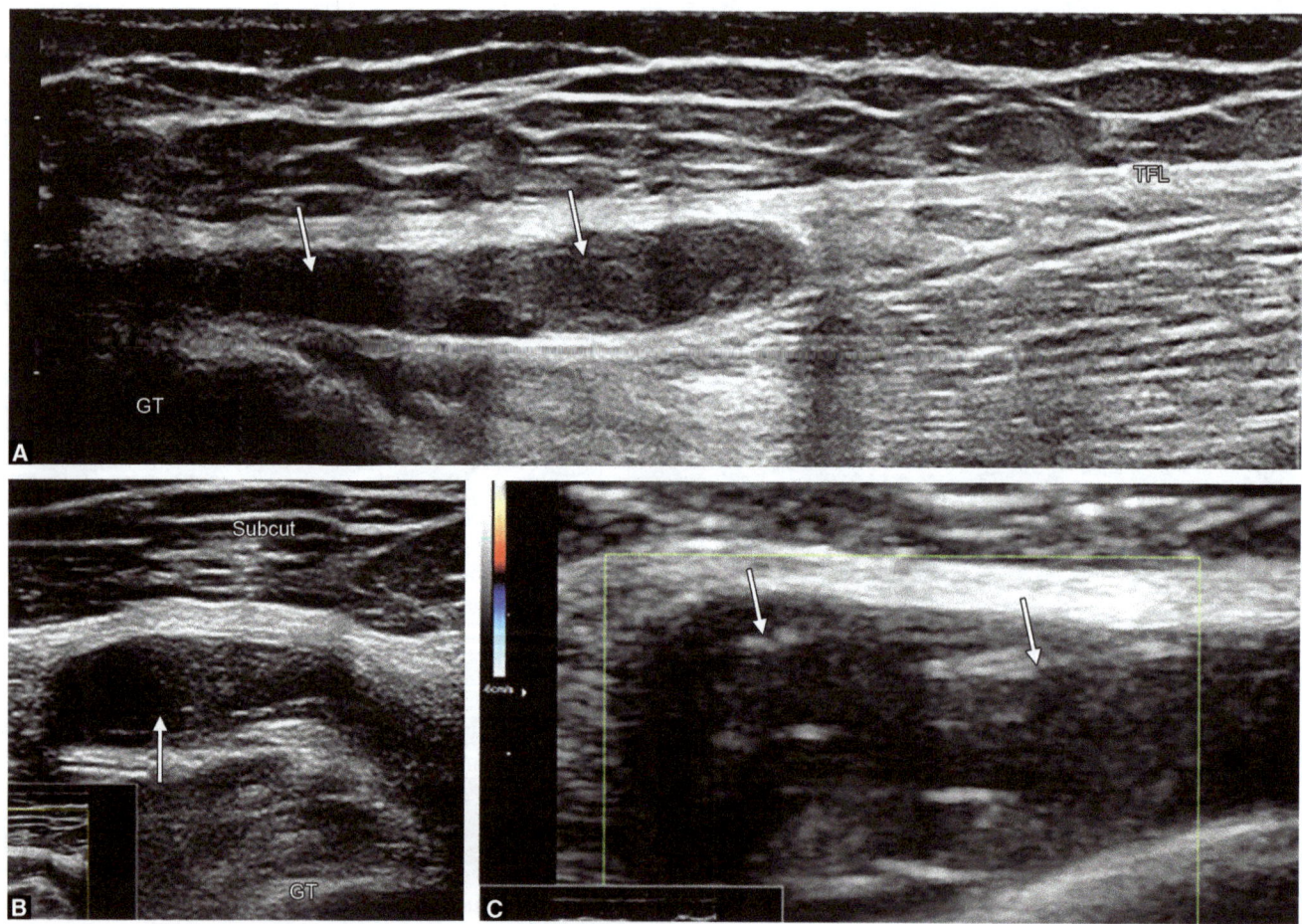

Figs. 1A to C: The distended greater trochanteric bursa (arrows) is seen as a cystic structure between the greater trochanter (GT) and the tensor fascia lata (TFL). Low-level internal echoes within the bursa (A and B) suggest synovial hypertrophy. Power Doppler (C) does not show any significant vascularity within the thickened bursa (arrows). (Subcut: Subcutaneous fat)

■ DIAGNOSIS

Greater trochanteric bursitis.

■ DISCUSSION

- The greater trochanteric bursa (GTB) is an anatomical bursa along the lateral aspect of the hip, covering the posterior facet of the greater trochanter. It is located beneath the gluteus maximus muscle and iliotibial tract.[1]
- Greater trochanteric pain syndrome is characterized by chronic lateral hip pain associated with tenderness over the greater trochanter.[2,3] Common causes of greater trochanteric pain syndrome include: (1) greater trochanteric bursitis, (2) gluteus medius tendinopathy, and (3) snapping hip.
- Impingement of the GTB against the fascia lata results in primary inflammation of the GTB. This mechanism is analogous to shoulder impingement.
- Inflammation of the GTB may occur due to other etiologies like crystal deposition disease, inflammatory arthropathies, connective tissue disease, and infections.
- *Ultrasound (US) findings in inflammation of the GTB are*:
    - Ill-defined edema over the greater trochanter
    - Effusion within the GTB with or without synovial hypertrophy
    - Calcification within the GTB
    - Power Doppler may or may not show neovascularity
    - Underlying tendinosis of the gluteus medius tendon (if any).
- Ultrasound-guided injection of corticosteroid may be done within the inflamed GTB.

■ REFERENCES

1. Horcajadas AB, Lafuente JL, de la Cruz Burgos R, et al. Ultrasound and MR findings in tumor and tumor-like lesions of the fingers. Eur Radiol. 2003;13:672-85.
2. Kingzett-Taylor A, Tirman PF, Feller J, et al. Tendinosis and tears of the gluteus medius and minimus muscles as a cause of hip pain: MR imaging findings. AJR Am J Roentgenol. 1999;173:1123-6.
3. Bass CJ, Connell DA. Sonographic findings of tensor fascia lata tendinopathy: another cause of anterior groin pain. Skeletal Radiol. 2002;31:143-8.

Case 53

Partial-thickness Tear of Gluteus Medius Tendon

■ CLINICAL HISTORY

A 51-year-old woman presented with pain along the lateral aspect of the right hip. The pain is exaggerated when she attempts to sit cross-legged. The patient is known to have diabetes mellitus.

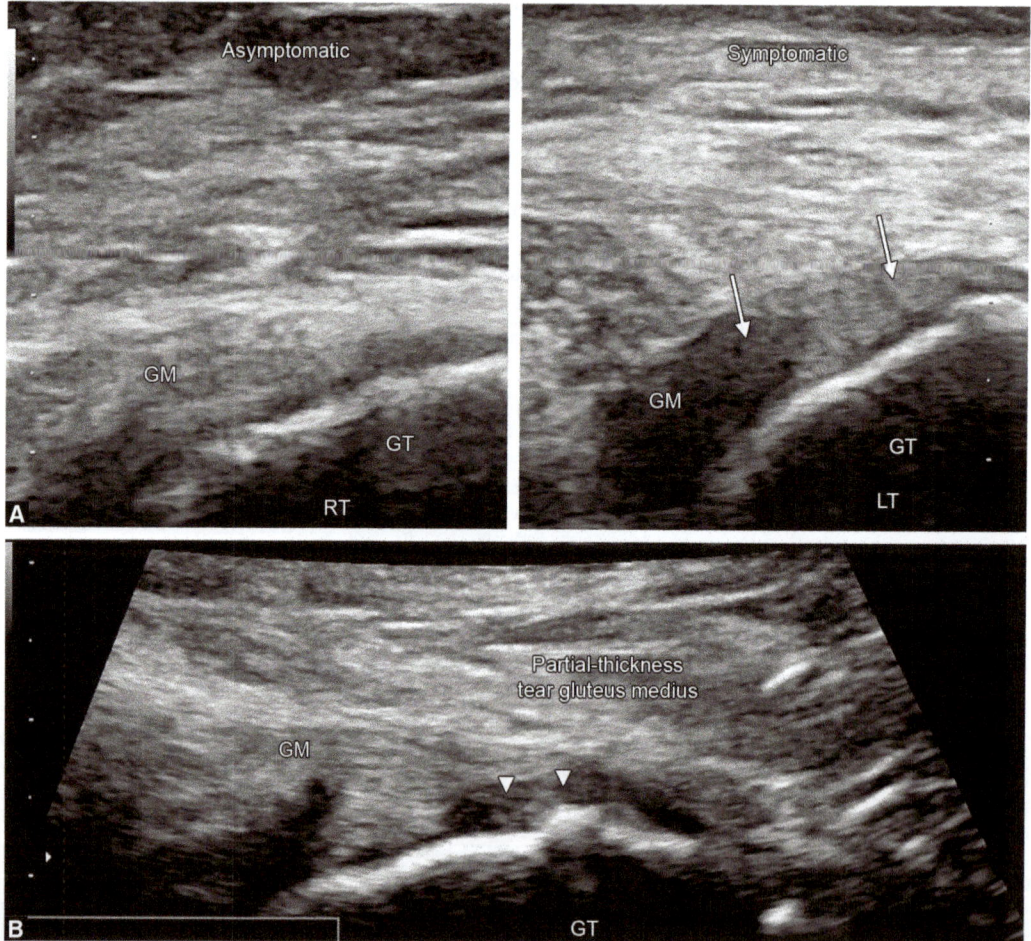

Figs. 1A and B: (A) Gluteus medius (GM) tendon of the symptomatic side appears diffusely thickened and hypoechoic compared to the asymptomatic side on the long-axis image; (B) Partial-thickness tear (arrowheads) of the GM tendon from its attachment over the greater trochanter (GT). (RT: right; LT: left)

DIAGNOSIS

Partial-thickness tear of the gluteus medius tendon.

DISCUSSION

- The gluteus medius and the gluteus minimus muscles are external rotators and abductors at the hip joint. The tendons of gluteus medius and gluteus minimus tendons fuse as they attach over the greater trochanter (GT). They are also known as "rotator cuff" of the lower limb.
- The gluteus minimus inserts over the anterior facet of the GT.
- While the main tendon of gluteus medius attaches to the superoposterior facet (of the GT), a broad attachment of the tendon is also seen over the lateral facet (Figs. 2A and B).
- The pathophysiology of inflammation of the gluteus medius tendon is similar to that of the greater trochanteric bursa, wherein the gluteus medius tendon gets impinged against the fascia lata.
- *Ultrasound findings in gluteus tendinopathy*:
    - Mild tendon enlargement
    - Hypoechoic appearance (Fig. 1A)
    - Partial-thickness/full-thickness tears (Fig. 1B)
    - Deep and anterior fibers of gluteus medius most commonly involved (Figs. 3 and 4)
    - Increased vascularity on power Doppler (uncommon)
    - Intratendinous calcification (Figs. 3 and 4)
    - Enthesopathic changes at the greater trochanter.

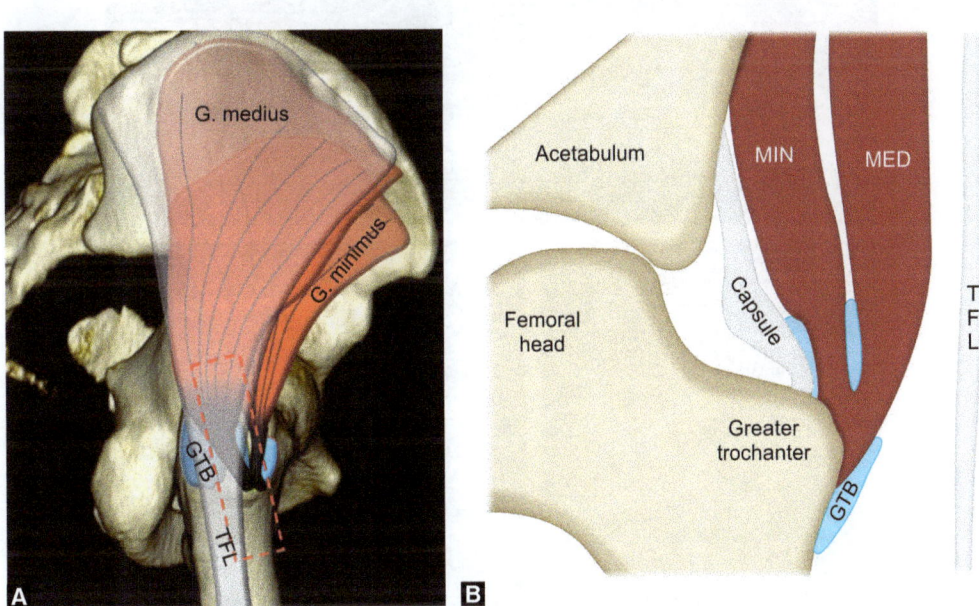

Figs. 2A and B: (A) Gluteus medius and gluteus minimus tendon insertion. Gluteus medius (G. medius) and gluteus minimus (G. minimus) tendons insert over the greater trochanter. The greater trochanteric bursa (GTB) covers the posterior facet of the greater trochanter (GT) and lies between the GT and tensor fascia lata (TFL). The red box in (A) shows the probe position; and (B) Diagrammatic representation of the gluteus tendons on the long-axis image. (MIN: minimus; MED: medius)

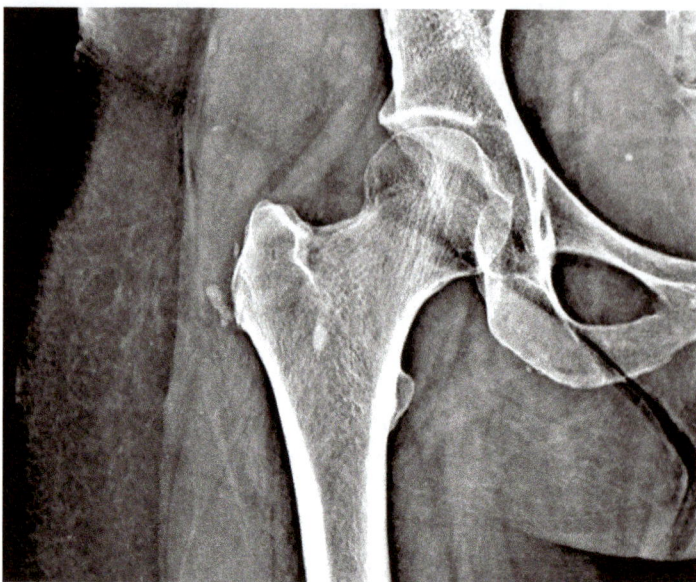

Fig. 3: The frontal radiograph shows nodular soft tissue calcification over the greater trochanter.

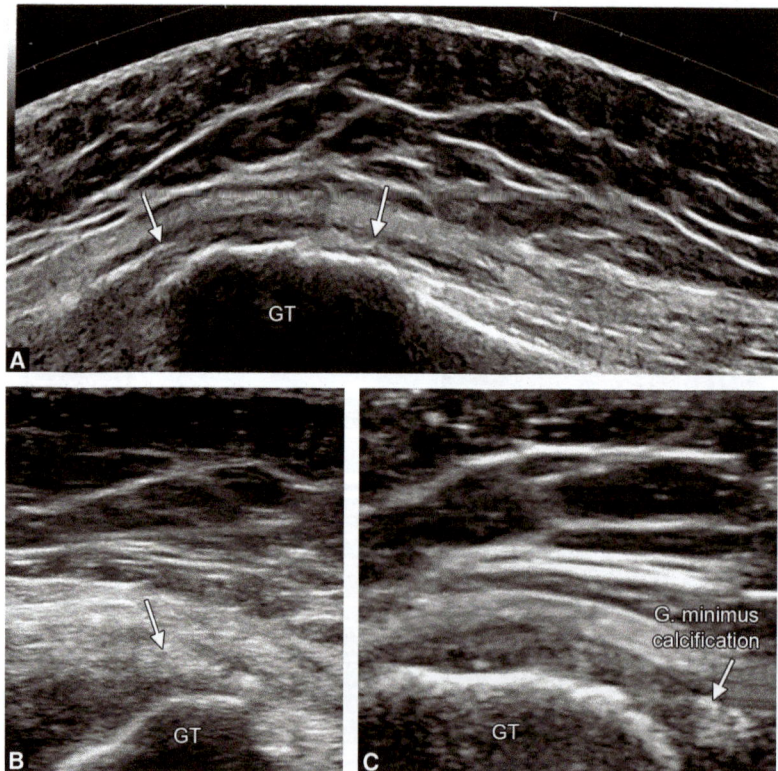

Figs. 4A to C: (A) Long-axis image immediately over the greater trochanter (GT) shows mild effusion in the greater trochanteric bursa (arrows); and (B and C) Long-axis and transverse images over the anterior facet of the GT show intratendinous calcification (arrows) within the gluteus minimus tendon. (G. minimus: gluteus minimus)

CASE 54

High-grade Partial Thickness Hamstring Tear with Hematoma

■ CLINICAL HISTORY

A 52-year-old man presented with a painful erythematous swelling along the posterior aspect of the left thigh following fall (Fig. 1).

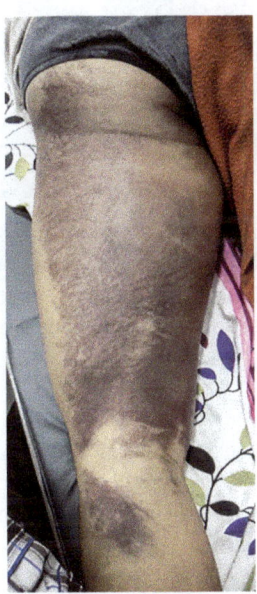

Fig. 1: Ill-defined swelling seen along the posterior aspect of the thigh with ecchymosis.

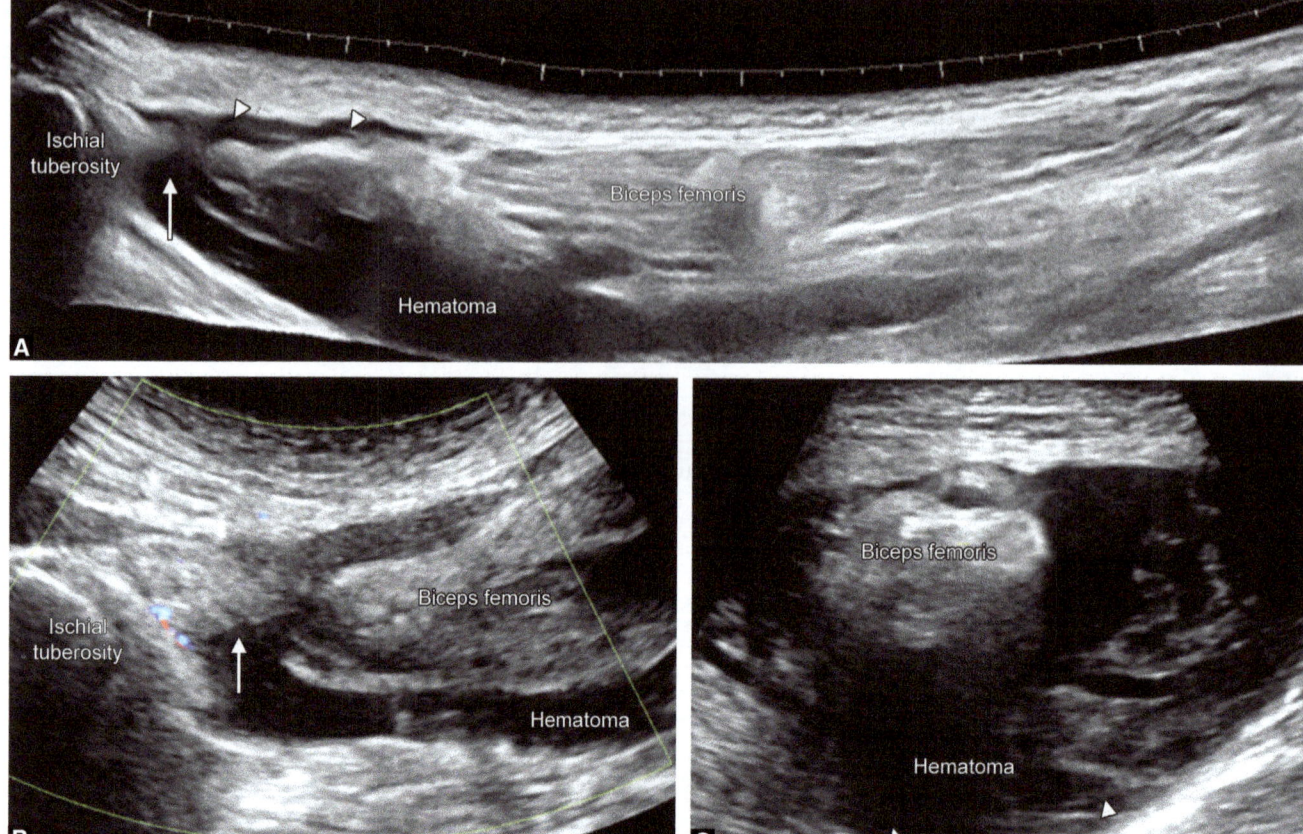

Figs. 2A to C: (A and B) Long axis images show a partial-thickness tear (arrows) of the hamstring group of tendons. The tear predominantly involves biceps femoris tendon; and (C) The torn edges appear irregular and are retracted distally. The defect caused due to the tear, is occupied by large hematoma (arrowheads in A and C).

■ DIAGNOSIS

High-grade tear of the hamstring tendons (biceps femoris) from its proximal attachment.

■ DISCUSSION

- Hamstring complex consists of three muscles: (1) semitendinosus, (2) biceps femoris (long head), and (3) semimembranosus.
- The hamstrings tendons take their origin from the ischial tuberosity. The long head of biceps femoris and the semitendinosus arise from a common tendon along the posteromedial aspect of the ischial tuberosity.[1]
- Hamstring injuries primarily occur due to eccentric stretching of the muscles, i.e. the muscle contracts the same time that it is being lengthened.[2]
- *Role of imaging in evaluation of hamstring injuries*:
    - Confirmation of clinical diagnosis
    - Assessment of the location and extent of tear
    - Assessment of longitudinal length of strain
    - To determine an osseous avulsion injury.

- *Ultrasound findings in hamstring injuries*:
  - Loss of pennate pattern
  - Edema
  - Muscle retraction
  - Hematoma
  - Calcification along torn edges—chronic injuries.

REFERENCES

1. Williams PL, Bannister LH, Berry MH, et al. Gray's Anatomy, 38th edition. New York: Churchill Livingstone; 1995.
2. Shellock FG, Fukunaga T, Mink JH, et al. Exertional muscle injury: evaluation of concentric versus eccentric actions with serial MR imaging. Radiology. 1991;179:659-64.

Case 55

Partial-thickness Tear of the Rectus Femoris with Hematoma

■ CLINICAL HISTORY

A 42-year-old professional athlete presented with pain and swelling along the anterior aspect of the thigh following hurdles race.

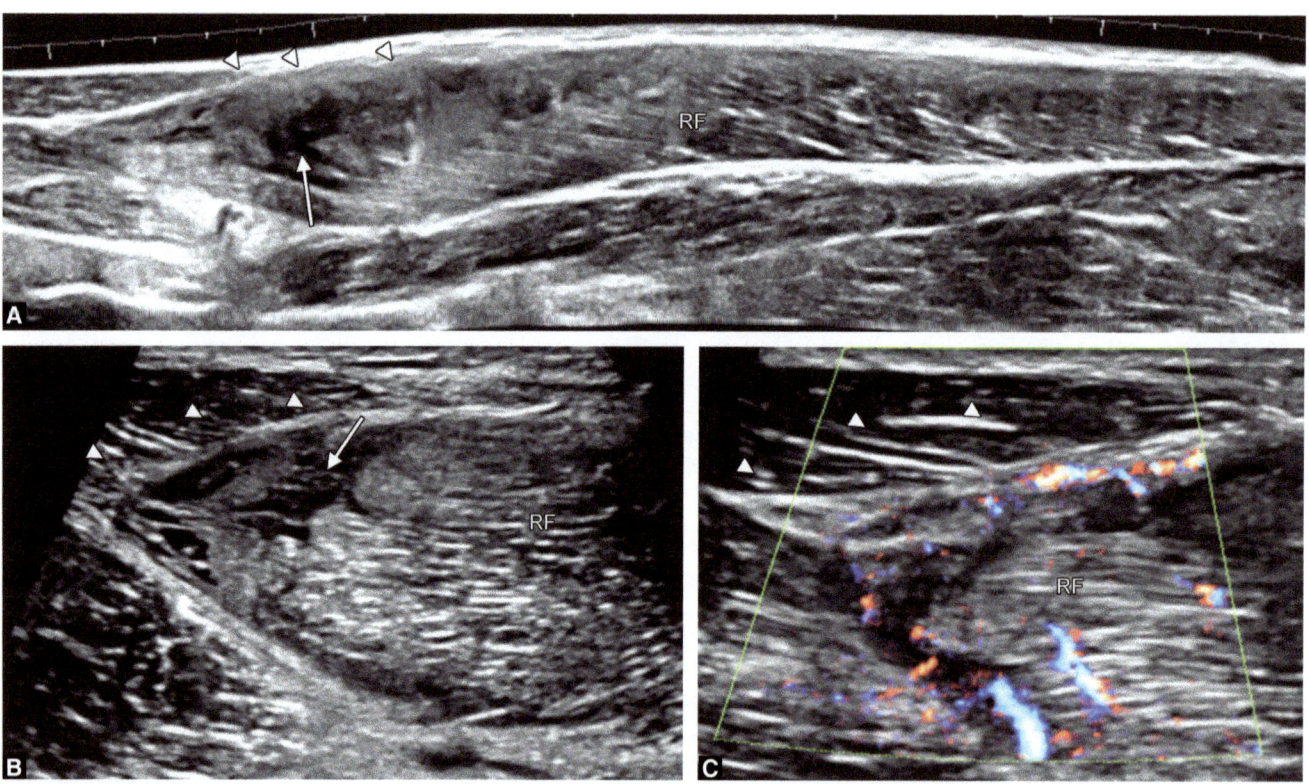

Figs. 1A to C: (A and B) Partial-thickness tear of the rectus femoris (RF) is seen as discontinuity of the muscle fibers (arrows) on long-axis and short-axis images. A hematoma is seen at the site of the tear; and (C) Power Doppler shows neovascularity along the torn margins. The arrowheads in A to C point to the muscle fascia.

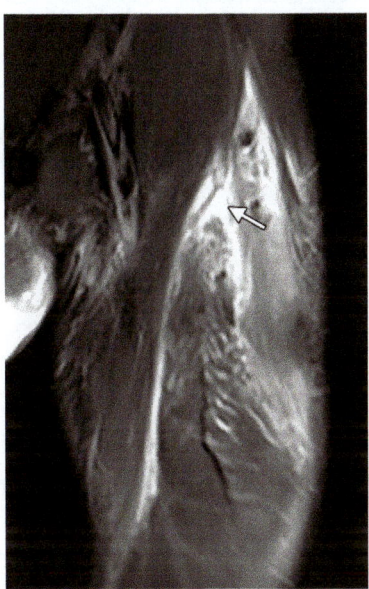

Fig. 2: Coronal T2 with fat-saturation MR imaging shows distal retraction of the partially torn rectus femoris muscle (arrow).

■ DIAGNOSIS

Partial-thickness tear of the rectus femoris tendon along the myo-aponeurotic junction with a hematoma.

Case 56

Acute Synovitis of the Right Hip

■ CLINICAL HISTORY

A 4-year-old boy presented with a limping gait and pain in the right hip since 2 days. There is no history of fever. White blood cell count was within normal range.

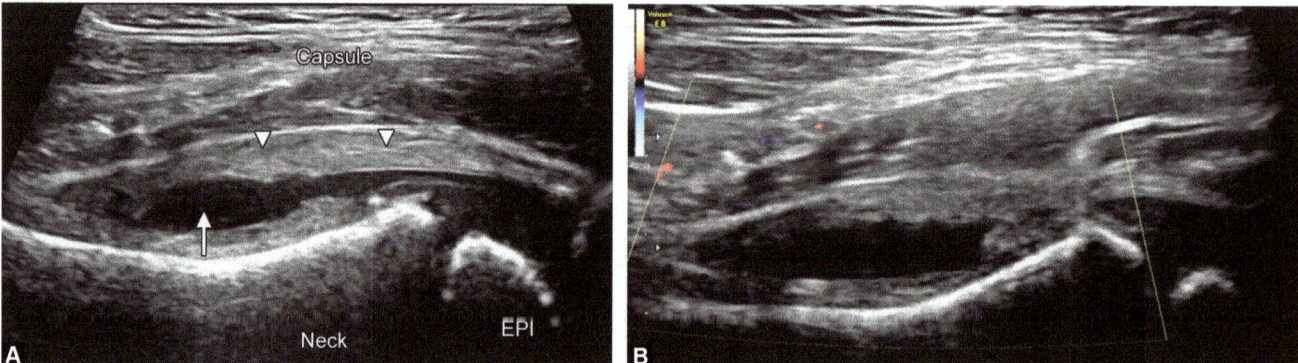

Figs. 1A and B: (A) Long-axis image of the hip shows mild effusion (arrow) in the anterior joint recess without any synovial hypertrophy. The effusion is seen to displace the joint capsule (arrowheads) anteriorly; and (B) Power Doppler does not show any vascularity within the joint recess. (EPI: epiphysis)

■ DIAGNOSIS

Acute synovitis of the right hip.

Case 57

Prepatellar Bursitis

CLINICAL HISTORY

A 64-year-old woman presented with swelling along the anterior aspect of the knee since 3 months.

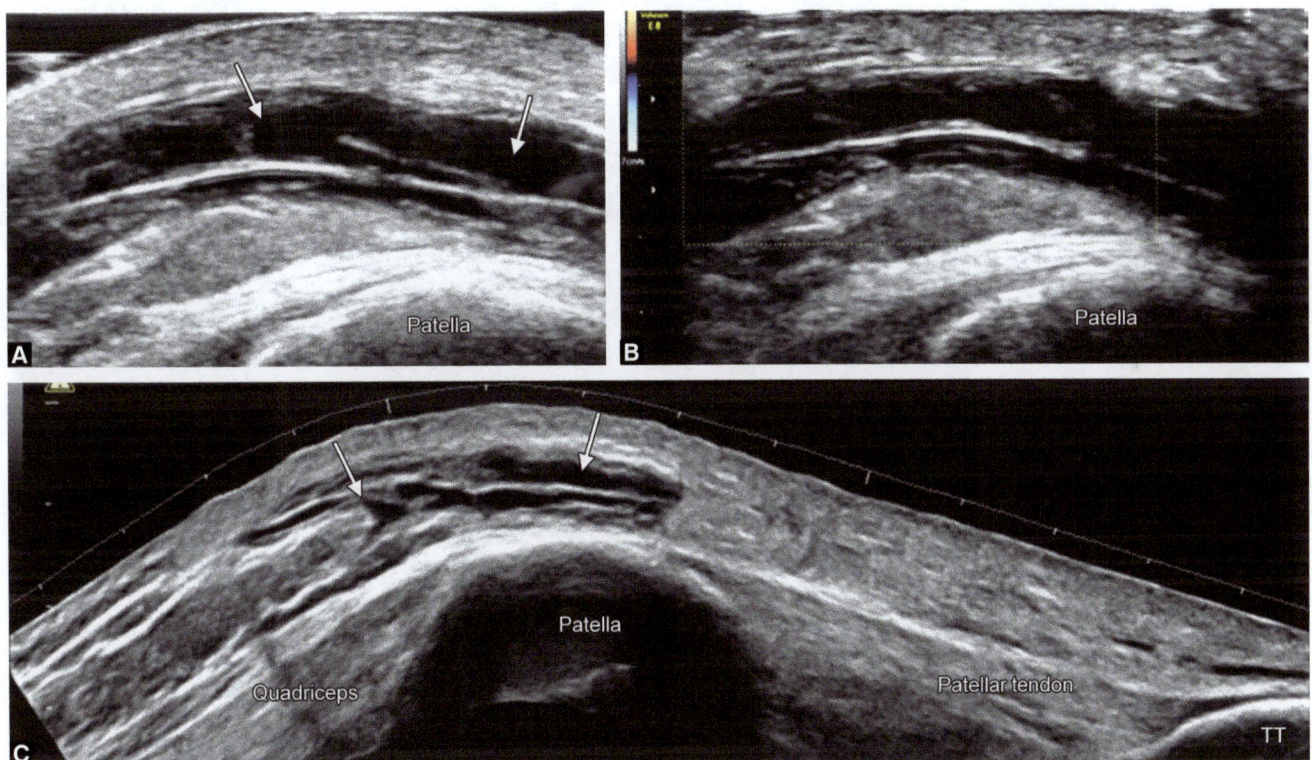

Figs. 1A to C: The distended prepatellar bursa is seen as a complex cystic structure (arrows) interposed between the subcutaneous fat and the anterior cortex of the patella. Few intralesional septae are also seen. Power Doppler does not show any intralesional vascularity. (TT: tibial tuberosity)

DIAGNOSIS

Prepatellar bursitis.

DISCUSSION

- Prepatellar bursa is an anatomical bursa located between the skin and the patella.
- Prepatellar bursa, superficial infrapatellar bursa, and deep infrapatellar bursa are the anatomical bursae, which are located along the anterior aspect of the knee (Fig. 3). The suprapatellar bursa is technically a recess of the knee joint.
- Prepatellar bursal inflammation may be acute or chronic depending on the nature of the etiology.

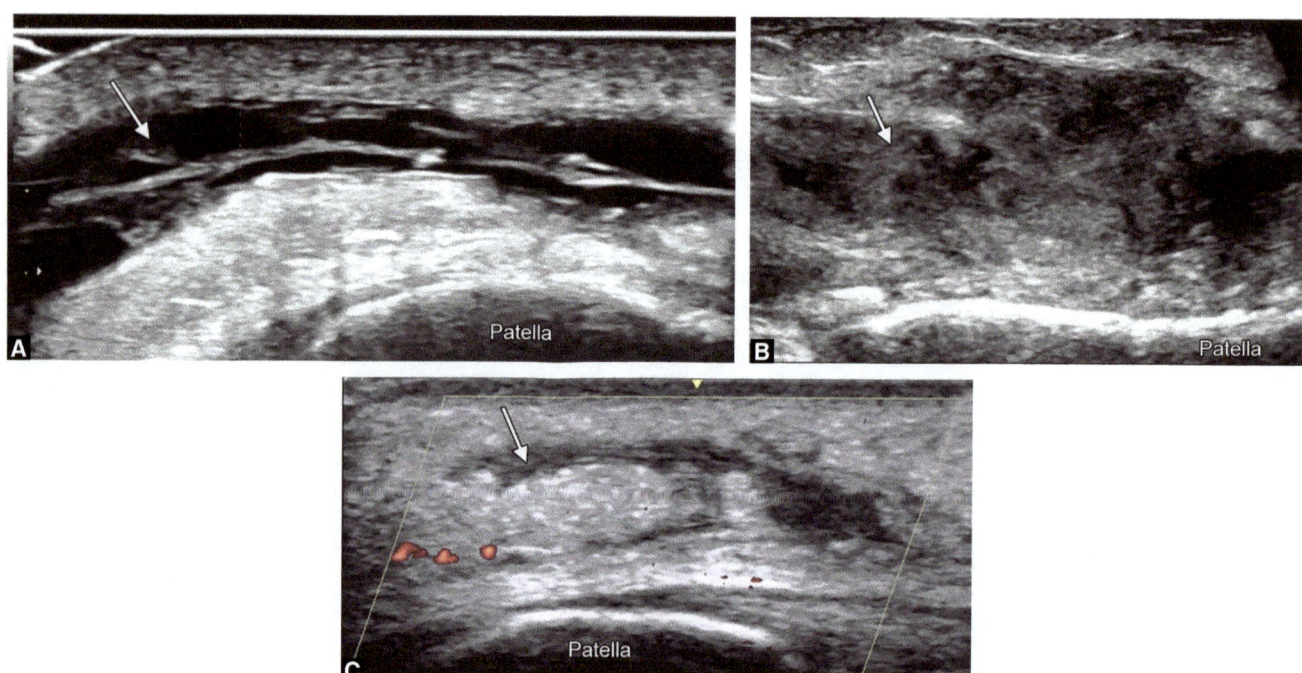

Figs. 2A to C: (A) Bursal thickening following acute trauma (arrow); (B) Bursal thickening with synovial hypertrophy in a known case of rheumatoid arthritis (arrow); and (C) Bursal thickening due to crystal deposition disease (arrow).

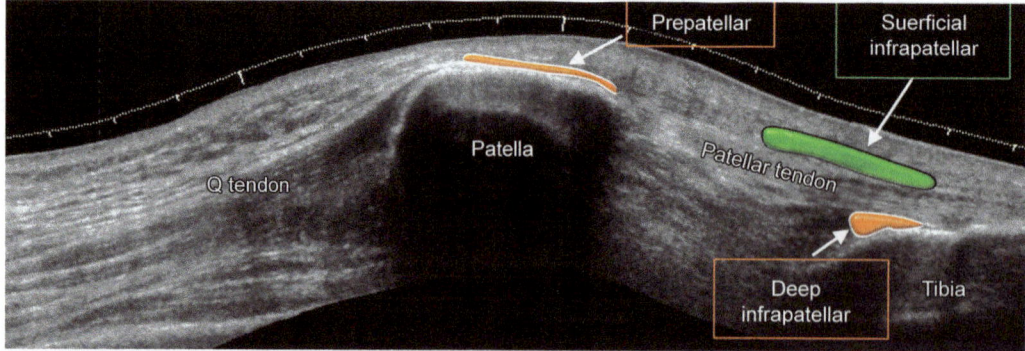

Fig. 3: Common bursae along the anterior aspect of the knee. (Q tendon: quadriceps tendon)

- *Ultrasound (US) features of prepatellar bursitis:*
  - Anechoic intrabursal fluid
  - Hemorrhagic bursa may present with echogenic intrabursal fluid
  - Chronic bursitis may have thick walls. Internal septations may or may not be present (Fig. 2A)
  - Synovial hypertrophy (Fig. 2B)
  - Neovascularity on power Doppler (Fig. 2C).
- *Role of US in imaging of bursal pathologies about the knee:*
  - Evaluation of bursal contents (fluid vs synovium)
  - Needle guidance for diagnostic and therapeutic aspiration
  - Intrabursal injection of corticosteroids.

Case 58

Superficial Infrapatellar Bursitis

■ CLINICAL HISTORY

A 22-year-old boy presented with a painful swelling along the anterior aspect of the knee.

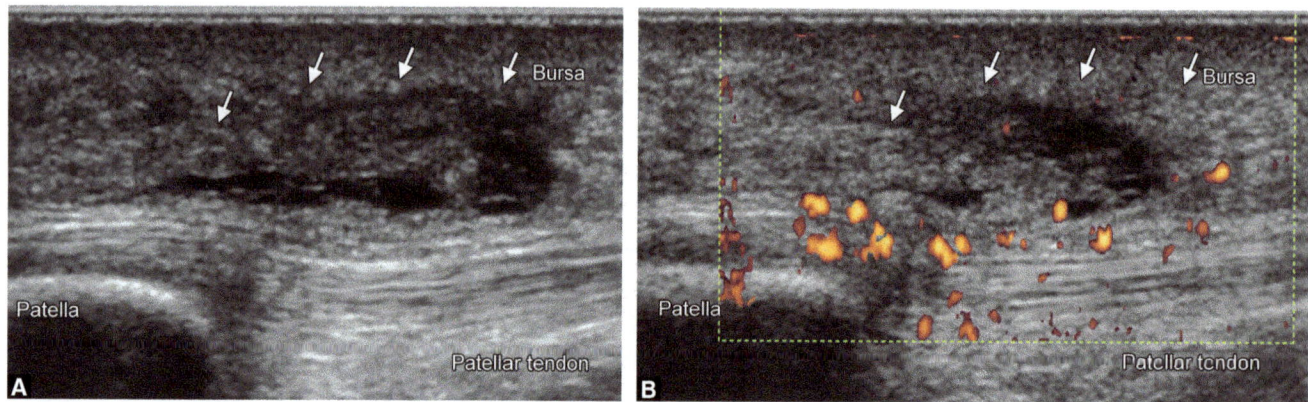

Figs. 1A and B: (A) Thickening of the prepatellar bursa (arrows) due to synovial hypertrophy and effusion; and (B) Power Doppler shows evidence of active inflammation in the form of increased vascularity.

■ DIAGNOSIS

Superficial infrapatellar bursitis.

ADDITIONAL CASE
■ HEMORRHAGIC SUPERFICIAL INFRAPATELLAR BURSITIS

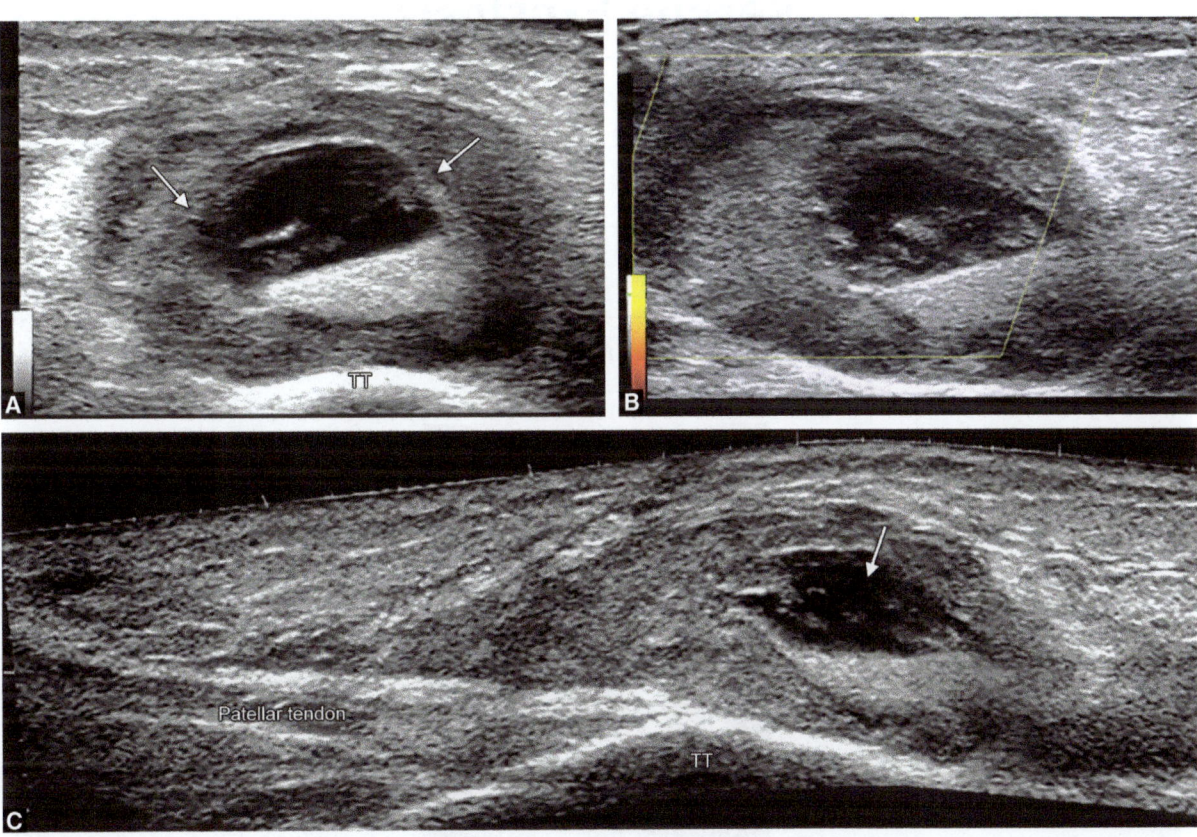

Figs. 2A to C: Effusion with fluid-fluid levels (arrows) within the enlarged superficial infrapatellar bursa. Power Doppler does not show any significant intralesional vascularity. (TT: tibial tuberosity)

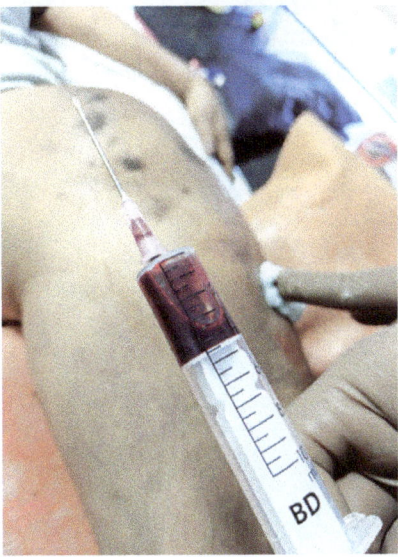

Fig. 3: Aspiration of the bursal contents yielded blood.

Case 59

Sessile Exostosis

■ CLINICAL HISTORY

A 19-year-old male presented with a firm swelling along the anterior aspect of the distal thigh since 2 years.

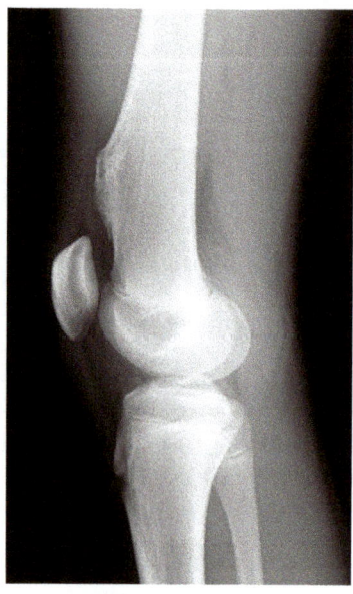

Fig. 1: Lateral radiograph of the knee shows a sessile exostosis arising from the anterior cortex of the distal femoral shaft.

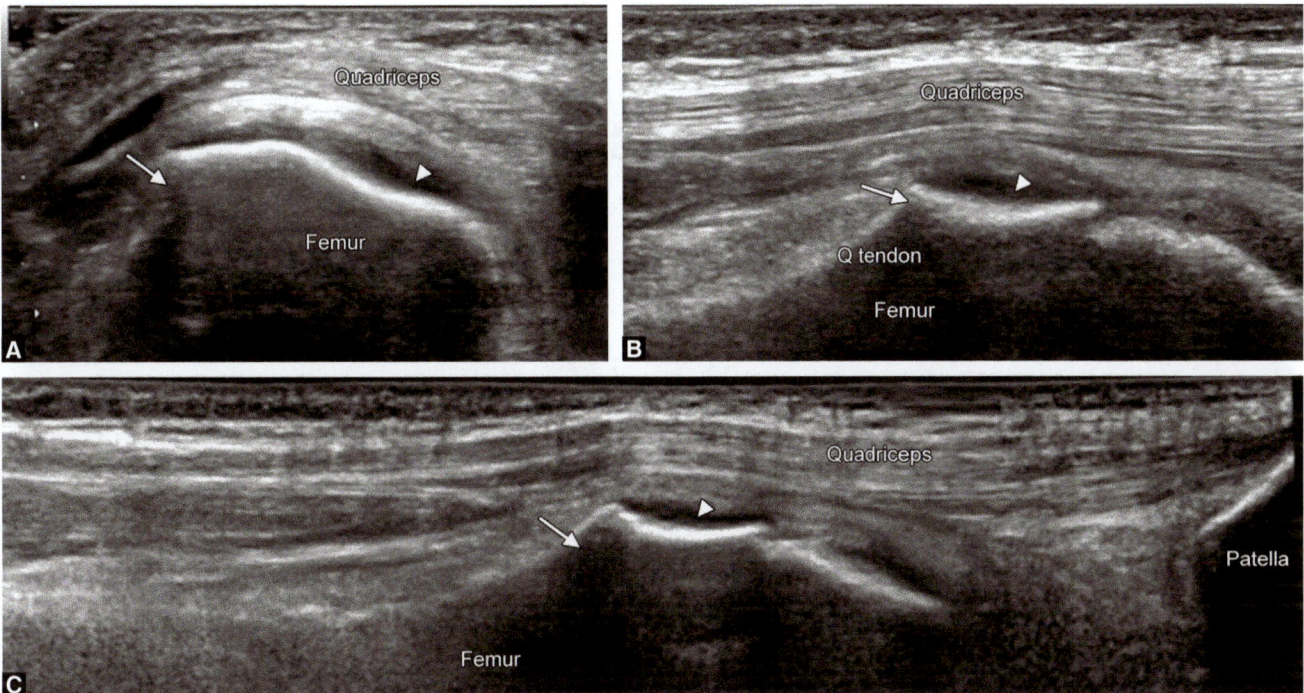

Figs. 2A to C: Transverse (A) and long-axis (B and C) images show smooth cortex of the exostosis (arrows). The cartilage cap is seen as a hypoechoic layer (arrowheads) overlying the exostosis. (Q tendon: quadriceps tendon)

DIAGNOSIS

Sessile exostosis.

DISCUSSION

- Exostosis is primarily diagnosed on radiographs (Fig. 1).
- Ultrasound (US) is primarily used to assess the cartilage thickness over the exostosis.
- On US, the cartilage is seen as a hypoechoic layer covering the echogenic cortex (Figs. 2A to C).
- Cartilage cap thickness of more than 2 cm is suspicious for malignant transformation.[1]

REFERENCE

1. Stephanie AB, Mark DM, Donald JF, et al. Improved differentiation of benign osteochondromas from secondary osteochondromas with standardized measurement of cartilage cap at CT and MR imaging. Radiology. 2010;255:857-65.

Case 60

Jumper's Knee

■ CLINICAL HISTORY

A 23-year-old volleyball player complained of anterior knee pain since 1 week. The pain was aggravated when he attempted to jump.

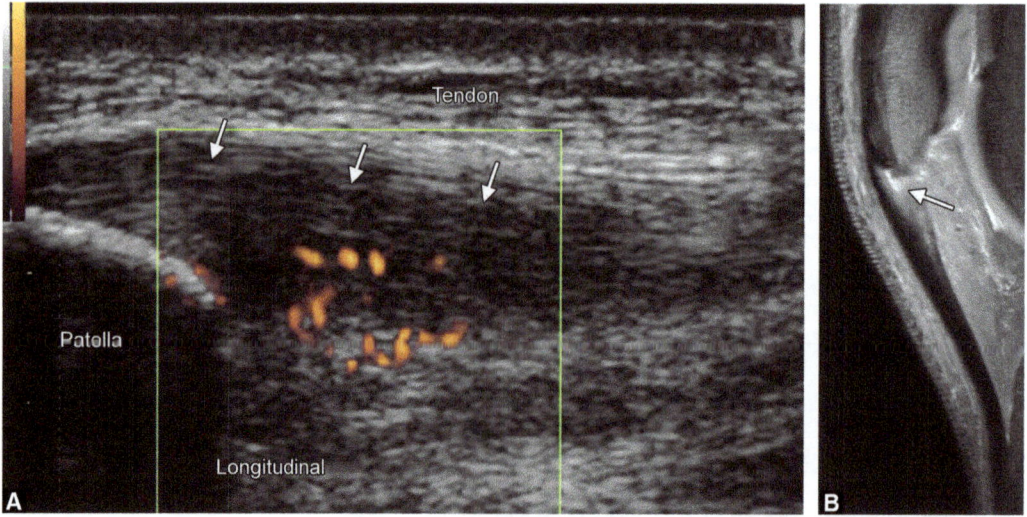

Figs. 1A and B: (A) Long-axis image shows inflammation of the deep fibers (arrows) of the patellar tendon close to its patellar attachment. Power Doppler shows significant vascularity within the tendon; and (B) Sagittal proton density with fat saturation MR image intratendinous T2 signal in the proximal patellar tendon (arrow).

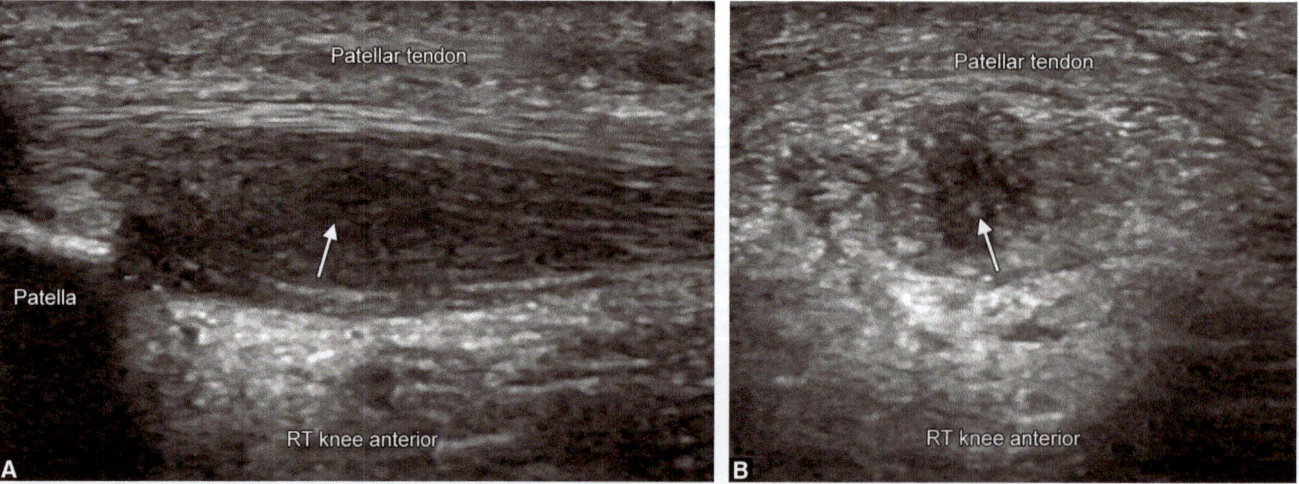

Figs. 2A and B: Long-axis and transverse images show focal inflammation of the proximal patellar tendon. The involved segment of the tendon appears diffusely thickened and hypoechoic (arrows). (RT: right)

DIAGNOSIS

Focal tendinosis of the patellar tendon at the upper pole of the patella (Jumper's knee).

DISCUSSION

- Inflammation of the patellar tendon commonly occurs close to its patellar attachment. The underlying mechanism is chronic microtrauma to the tendon.
- *Role of ultrasound (US)*:
    - To confirm clinical diagnosis
    - To differentiate tendinosis versus tear
    - Focal versus diffuse
    - To assess the extent and severity of the pathology.
- *USG findings in patellar tendinosis and tear*:
    - Peri-insertional fusiform hypoechoic area (Figs. 1A and B)
    - Deep central portion (Figs. 2A and B)
    - Focal hyperechoic spots and shadowing
    - Posterior bulging tendon
    - Increased vascularity in chronic tendinosis
    - Partial tear—anechoic area/complete tear—discontinuity of fibers
    - Follow-up.

Case 61

Full-thickness Tear of the Patellar Tendon

CLINICAL HISTORY

A 31-year-old man presented with inability to extend the knee following road traffic accident.

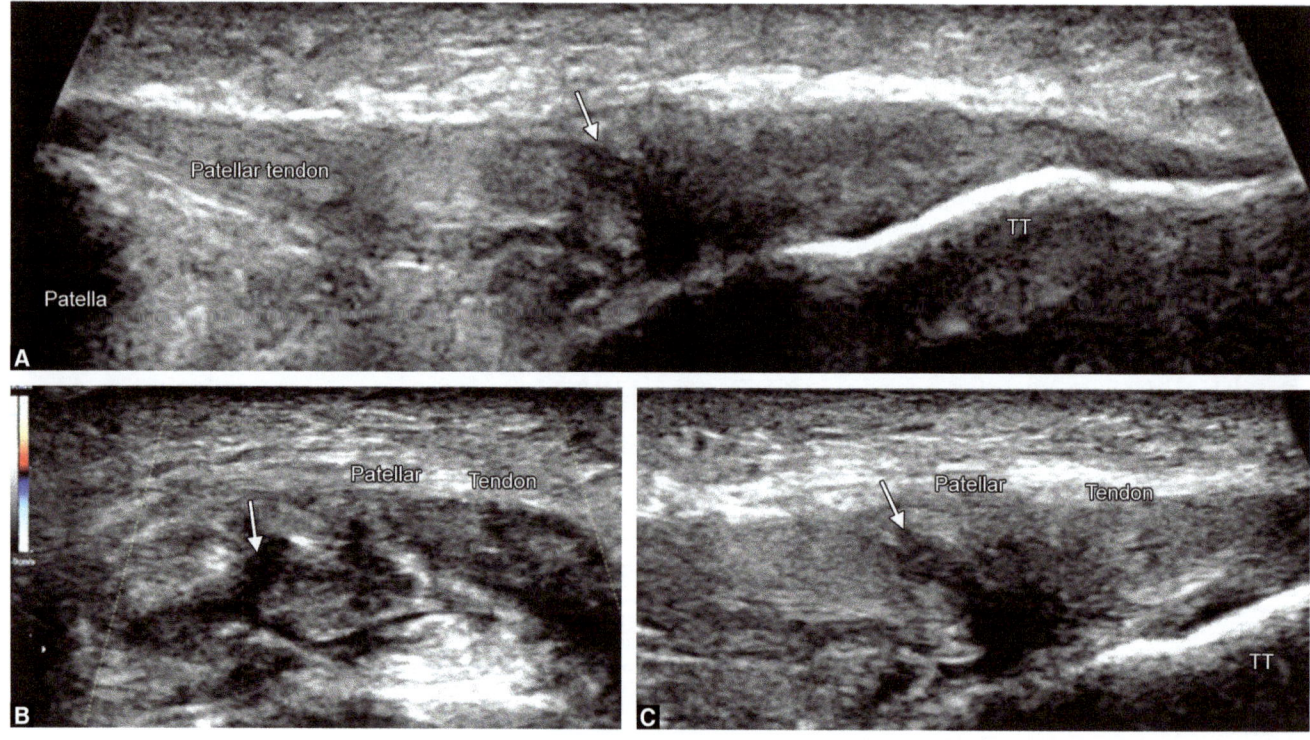

Figs. 1A to C: Long and short-axis images of the patellar tendon show discontinuity of the patellar tendon (arrows) suggestive of a complete full-thickness midsubstance tear. (TT: tendon tear)

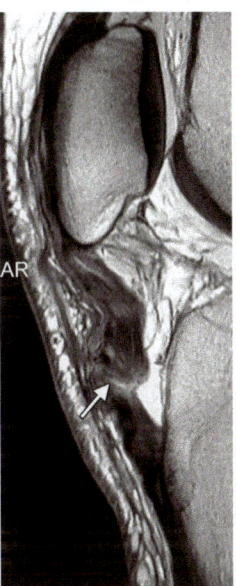

Fig. 2: Sagittal proton density MR image shows a full-thickness tear (arrow) of the patellar tendon.

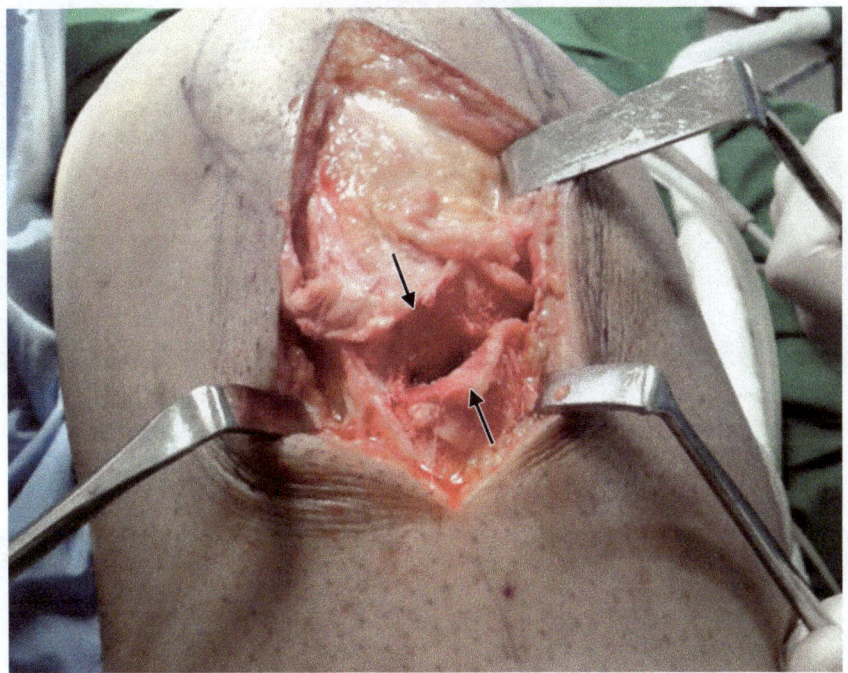

Fig. 3: Intraoperative image showing reflected edges (arrows) of the torn patellar tendon.

■ DIAGNOSIS

Full-thickness midsubstance tear of the patellar tendon.

Case 62

Full-thickness Tear of the Quadriceps Tendon

CLINICAL HISTORY

A 27-year-old male presented with acute pain and swelling along the anterior aspect of the knee after sustaining a fall during a game of football. There is loss of knee extension.

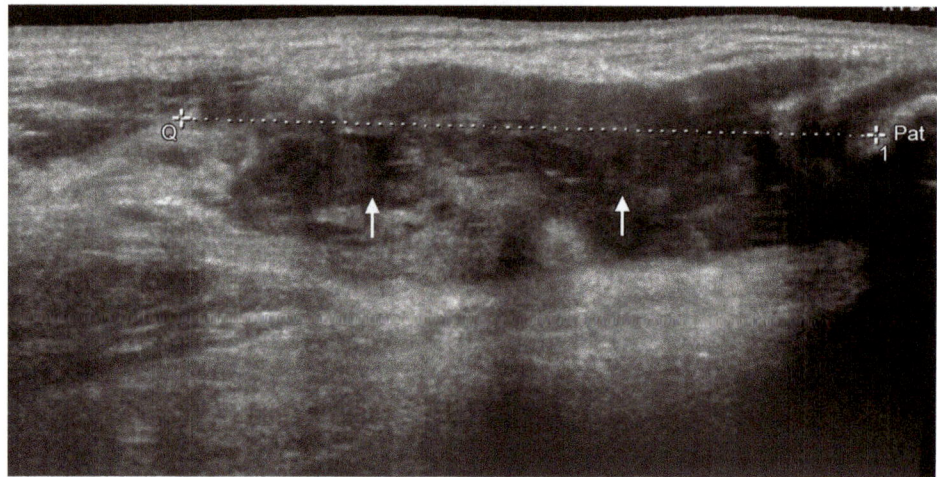

Fig. 1: Long-axis image shows a full-thickness tear (arrows) of the quadriceps tendon from the site of its patellar attachment. The margins of the retracted quadriceps tendon appear frayed. Extended field of view or panoramic imaging is quite useful in evaluation of the entire extent of the tear. (Pat: patella; Q: quadriceps tendon)

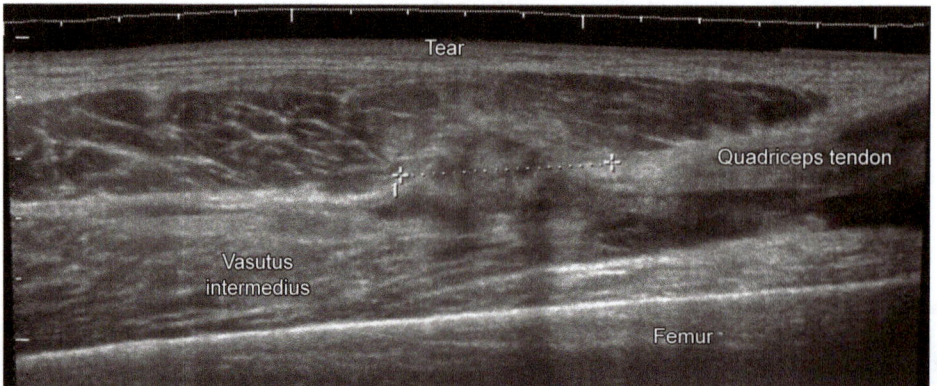

Fig. 2: Long-axis image shows a midsubstance tear of the quadriceps tendon close to the myoaponeurotic junction. An ill-defined hematoma is seen at the site of the tear.

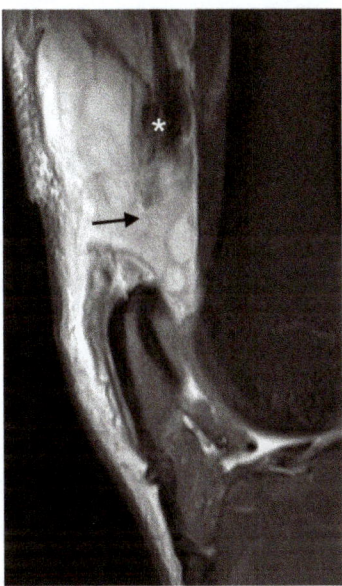

Fig. 3: Sagittal proton density with fat saturation MR image shows tear of the qadriceps (arrow) with proximally retracted torn margin of the tendon.
*Retracted quadriceps tendon

DIAGNOSIS

Full-thickness tear of the quadriceps tendon with proximal retraction of the torn edges.

DISCUSSION

- The quadriceps tendon and the patellar tendon form the extensor mechanism of the knee.[1] The quadriceps tendon has a striated appearance. Rectus femoris forms the superficial layer of the quadriceps tendon. Middle layer of the quadriceps tendon is formed by tendons of vastus medialis and the vastus lateralis. The deepest layer of quadriceps tendon is formed by vastus intermedius.[2]
- Spontaneous injuries of the quadriceps tendon are uncommon.
- Systemic risk factors for a tear of the quadriceps tendon include: gout, diabetes mellitus, chronic kidney disease, hyperparathyroidism, and rheumatoid arthritis.
- *Role of ultrasound (US)*:
    - Differentiation of partial thickness versus full-thickness tear
    - Percentage of tendon thickness involvement in the tear (Fig. 1)
    - Degree of proximal retraction of the torn tendon (Figs. 2 and 3)
    - Presence of osseous avulsion from the superior pole of patella
    - Dynamic examination
    - Ultrasound can evaluate the quadriceps tendon in the postoperative knee in the presence of metallic implants.

REFERENCES

1. Wangwinyuvirat M, Dirim B, Pastore D, et al. Prepatellar quadriceps continuation: MRI of cadavers with gross anatomic and histologic correlation. AJR Am J Roentgenol. 2009;192:W111-6.
2. Fulkerson JP. Disorders of the Patellofemoral Joint, 4th edition. Philadelphia: Lippincott Williams & Wilkins; 2004.

Case 63

Effusion in the Suprapatellar Recess

■ CLINICAL HISTORY

A 57-year-old man presented with chronic pain and swelling over the left knee. He had undergone an arthroplasty of the ipsilateral knee 7 months ago.

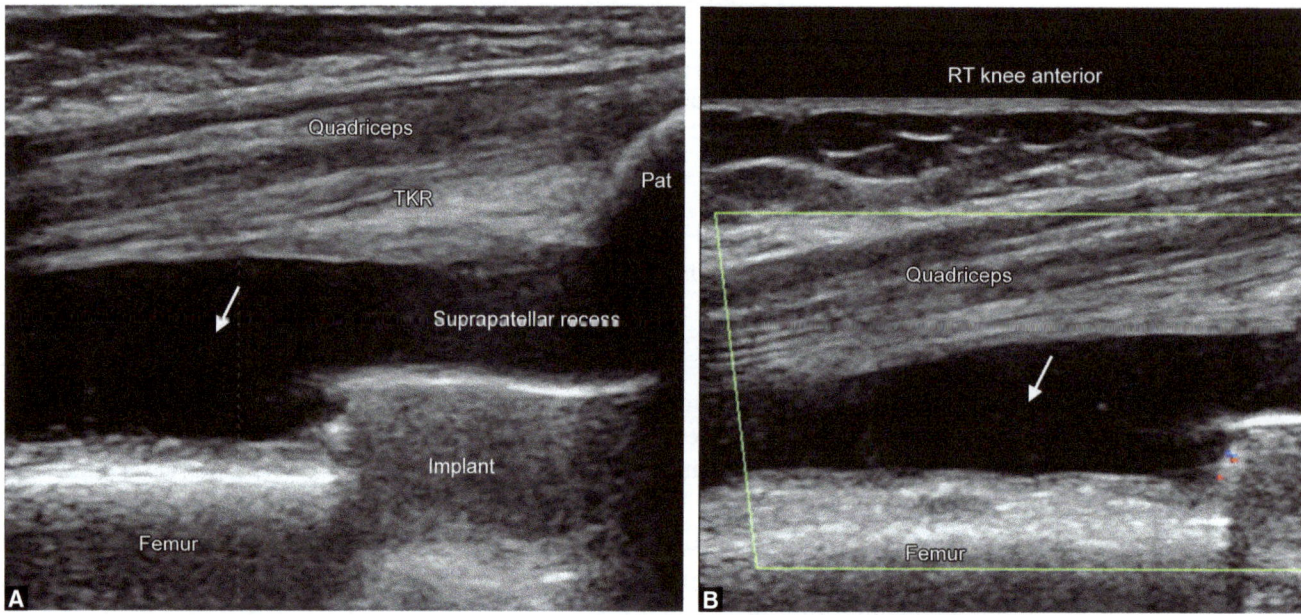

Figs. 1A and B: Long-axis images of the suprapatellar recess show moderate effusion (arrows) with few low-level internal echoes. There is no synovial hypertrophy or intra-articular vascularity of power Doppler images. There are no cortical erosions along the interface between the knee prosthesis and the distal femoral shaft. (TKR: total knee replacement; Pat: patella; RT: right)

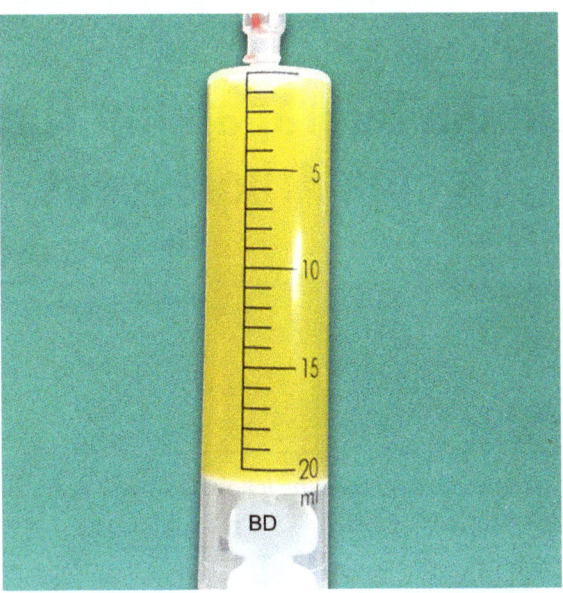

Fig. 2: Diagnostic aspiration of the knee yielded mildly turbid straw-colored fluid.

DIAGNOSIS

Moderate effusion in the suprapatellar recess with few low-level internal echoes. The patient subsequently underwent diagnostic aspiration of the knee which yielded exudative fluid (inflammation).

Case 64

Effusion in the Suprapatellar Recess with Lipoma Arborescens

■ CLINICAL HISTORY

A 75-year-old woman presented with chronic pain over the left knee since 2 years. Radiographs of the left knee showed mild reduction in the medial tibiofemoral joint space.

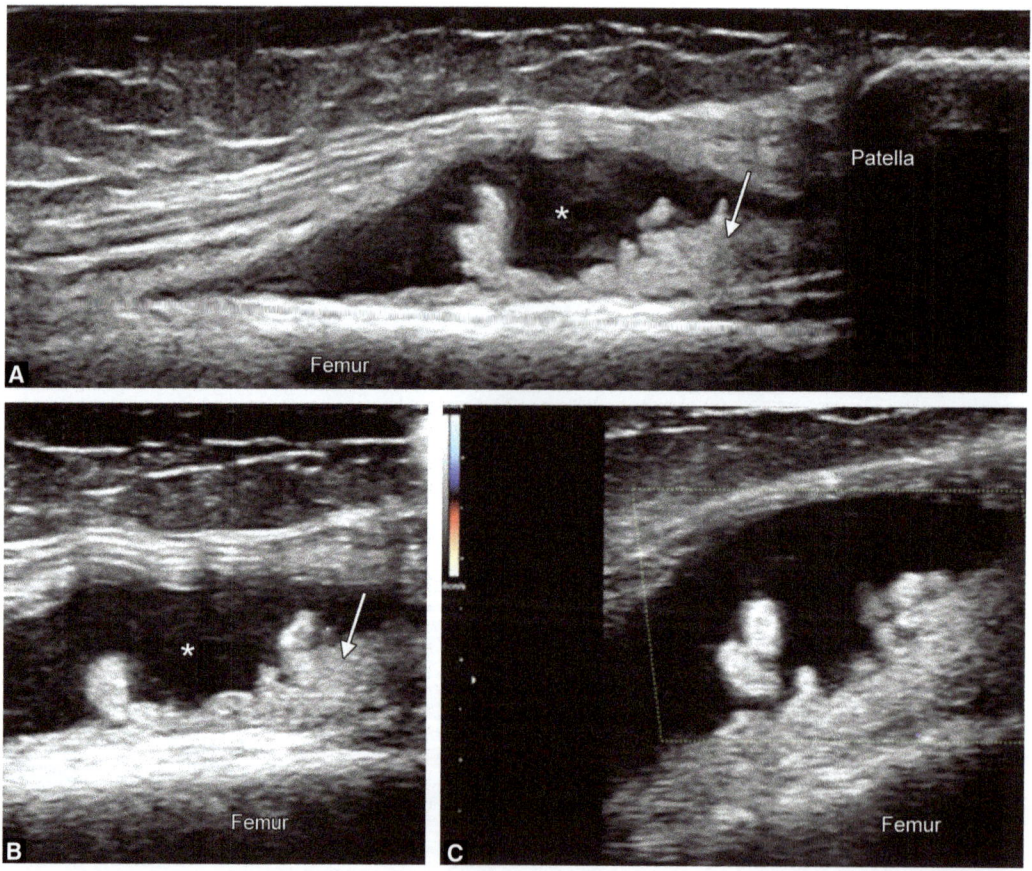

Figs. 1A to C: Moderate effusion (*) is seen in the suprapatellar recess with nodular hypertrophy of the synovium (arrows). The thickened synovium appears diffusely echogenic without any evidence of vascularity on power Doppler images.

■ DIAGNOSIS

Moderate effusion in the suprapatellar recess with lipoma arborescens.

Case 65

Baker's Cyst with Synovitis

CLINICAL HISTORY

A 42-year-old male presented with pain along the posteromedial aspect of the knee since 2 months. He is a known case of rheumatoid arthritis.

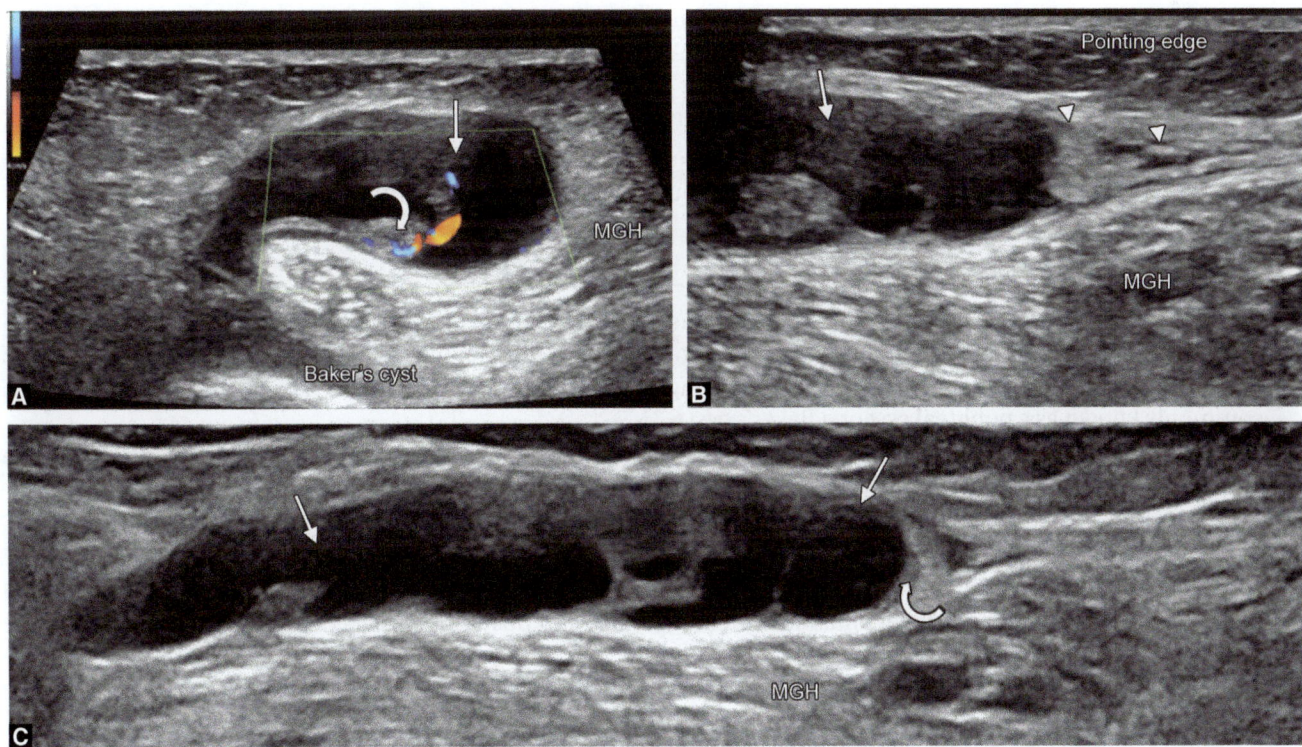

Figs. 1A to C: (A) Transverse and long-axis images of the Baker's cyst show synovial hypertrophy (curved arrows) along with neovascularity on color Doppler images; and (B and C) On long-axis images, the distal edge of the Baker's cyst appears pointed (arrowheads). Ill-defined edema is seen along the lower margin of the cyst. The arrows point to the effusion in the Baker's cyst. (MGH: medial gastrocnemius head)

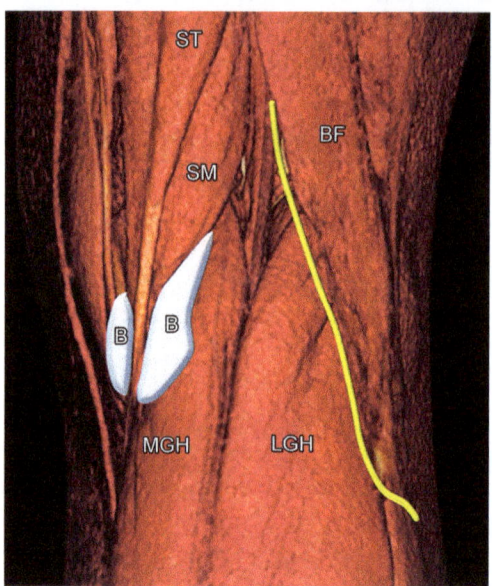

Fig. 2: Gastrocnemius-semimembranosus bursa. The gastrocnemius-semimembranosus bursa (B) is located between the medial gastrocnemius head (MGH) and the semimembranosus (SM). (BF: biceps femoris; LGH: lateral gastrocnemius head; ST: semitendinosus)

■ DIAGNOSIS

Effusion in the gastrocnemius-semimembranosus (GS) bursa with synovial hypertrophy.

■ DISCUSSION

- The GS bursa is located along the posteromedial aspect of the knee situated between the medial head of the gastrocnemius and the semimembranosus tendon (Fig. 2). The bursa may or may not communicate with the knee joint.
- The distended GS bursa is felt as a palpable lump along the posteromedial aspect of the knee. The distended bursa is commonly known as a popliteal cyst or a Baker's cyst.
- The contents of the knee (effusion, hemorrhage, loose bodies, and synovial hypertrophy) may extend into or involve the GS bursa.
- Idiopathic Baker's cyst may be seen in the pediatric age group.
- *Ultrasound features of Baker's cyst*:
    - Typical location along the posteromedial aspect of the knee. On transverse views, it is found in the triangle formed by the medial head of gastrocnemius, semimembranosus, and posterior surface of the medial femoral condyle (Figs. 1A to C)
    - The Baker's cyst typically demonstrates a base, neck, and body.
- *Contents of Baker's cyst*:
    - Simple fluid
    - Thick synovium
    - Caseous material
    - Loose bodies.
- *Complications of Baker's cyst*:
    - Rupture
    - Hemorrhage
    - Infection.

Case 66

Baker's Cyst

CLINICAL HISTORY

A 9-year-old girl presented a painless swelling along the posteromedial aspect of the knee.

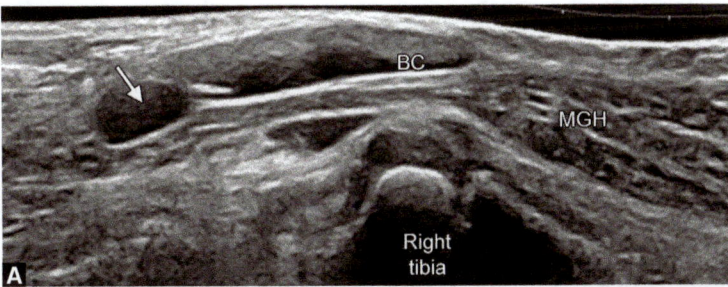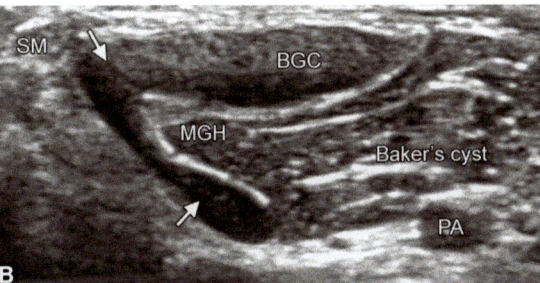

Figs. 1A and B: Long-axis and transverse images show the gastrocnemius-semimembranosus bursa (arrows) containing simple fluid. The bursa is located between the medial gastrocnemius head (MGH) and the semimembranosus (SM) muscle. The distended bursa is known as a Baker's cyst (BC). (PA: popliteal artery)

DIAGNOSIS

Baker's cyst.

Case 67

Tennis Leg

■ CLINICAL HISTORY

A 42-year-old male presented with acute pain and swelling along the posterior aspect of the calf with ecchymosis (Fig. 1).

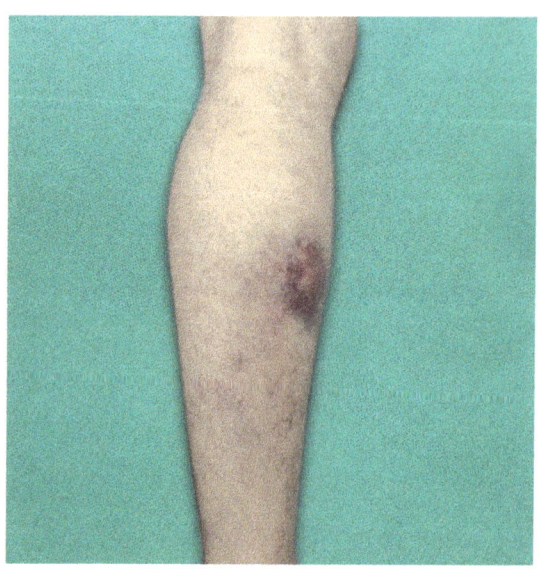

Fig. 1: Painful swelling along the medial aspect of the calf along with ecchymosis.

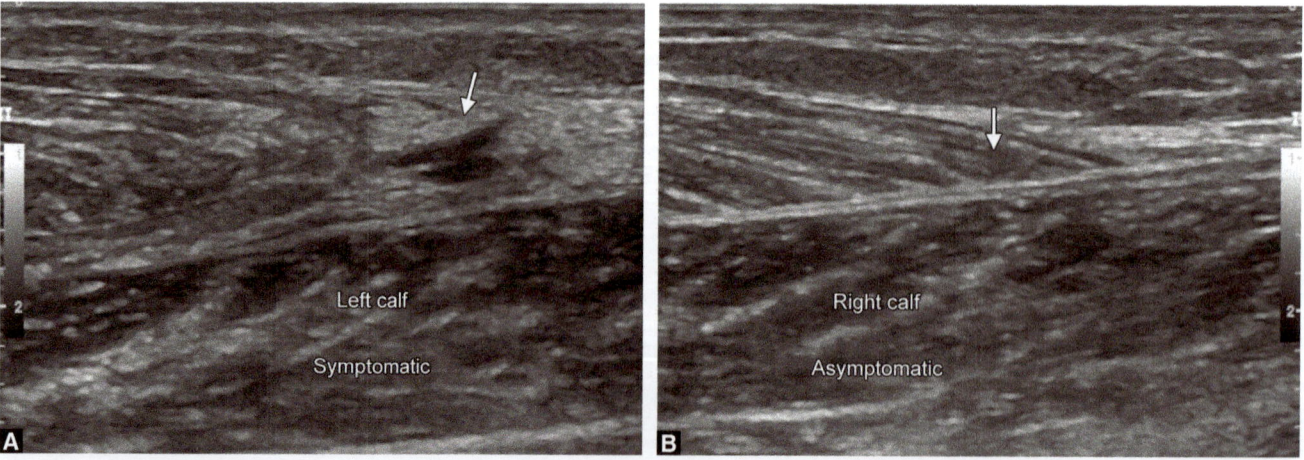

Figs. 2A and B: (A) Long-axis view of the affected calf shows a partial-thickness tear (arrow) of the medial head of the gastrocnemius at the myoaponeurotic junction. (B) Comparison with the asymptomatic side shows normal pennate pattern of the medial head of gastrocnemius (arrow).

■ DIAGNOSIS

Partial thickness tear of the medial head of gastrocnemius along the myoaponeurotic junction (tennis leg) (Figs. 2A and B).

■ DISCUSSION

Role of sonography in assessment of calf muscle injuries:
- To rule out deep venous thrombosis
- Differentiate between partial and complete tear (Figs. 3A to C)
- Dynamic examination allows assessment of the tear
- Size and extent of tear and muscle retraction
- Evaluate plantaris tendon.

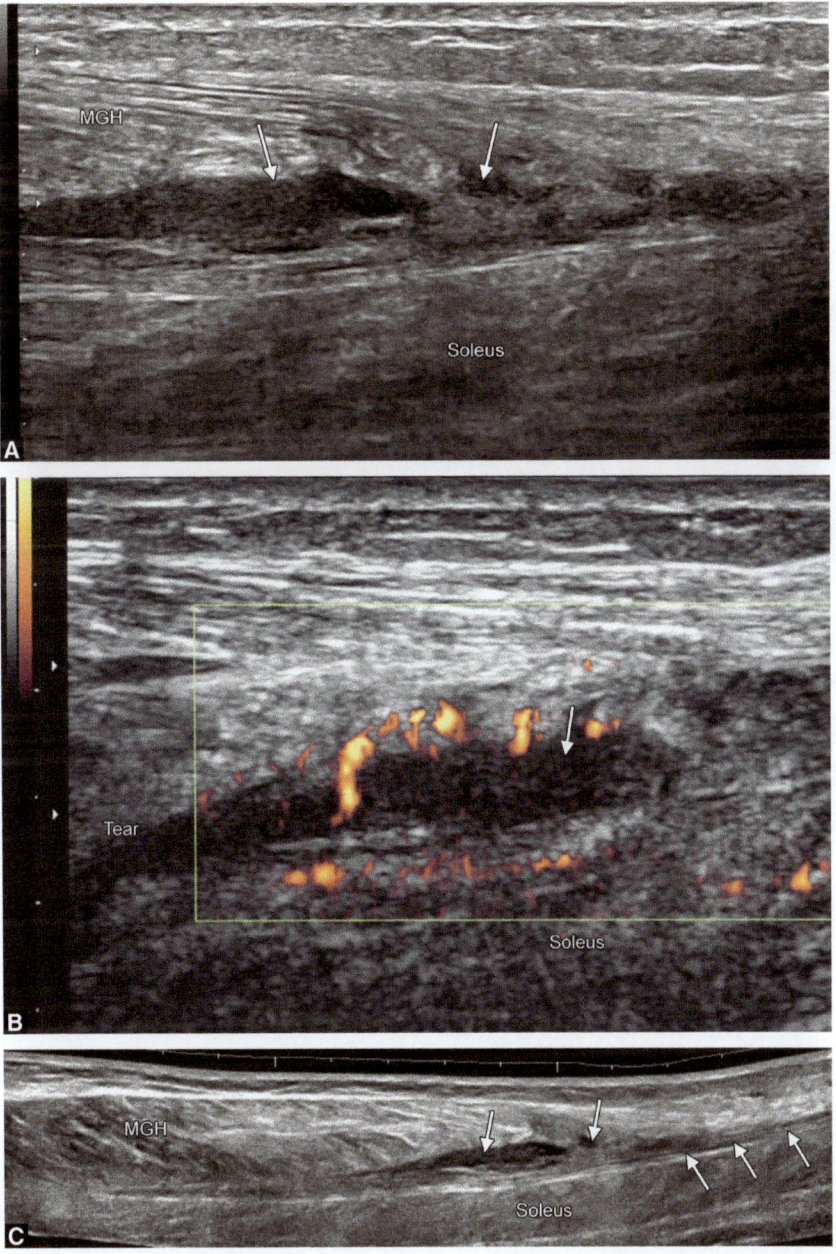

Figs. 3A to C: (A) Long-axis image shows a partial-thickness tear (arrows) of the medial head of the gastrocnemius (MGH) at the myoaponeurotic junction along with a hematoma; (B) Power Doppler shows increased vascularity along margins of the tear (arrow); (C) Extended field of view along the long axis of the calf demonstrates the entire extent of the calf tear (arrows). (MGH: medial gastrocnemius head)

Case 68

Herniation of the Tibialis Anterior Muscle

■ CLINICAL HISTORY

A 27-year-old factory worker presented with intermittent painless swelling along the anterior aspect of the left leg since 2 years. The swelling increased in size during squatting.

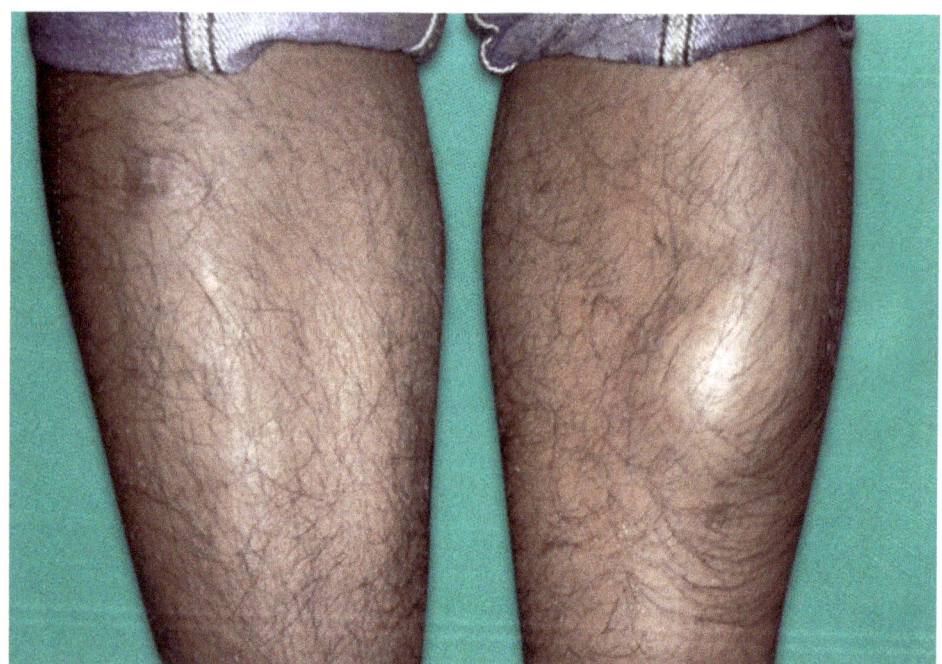

Fig. 1: Intermittent swelling along the anterior aspect of the left leg.

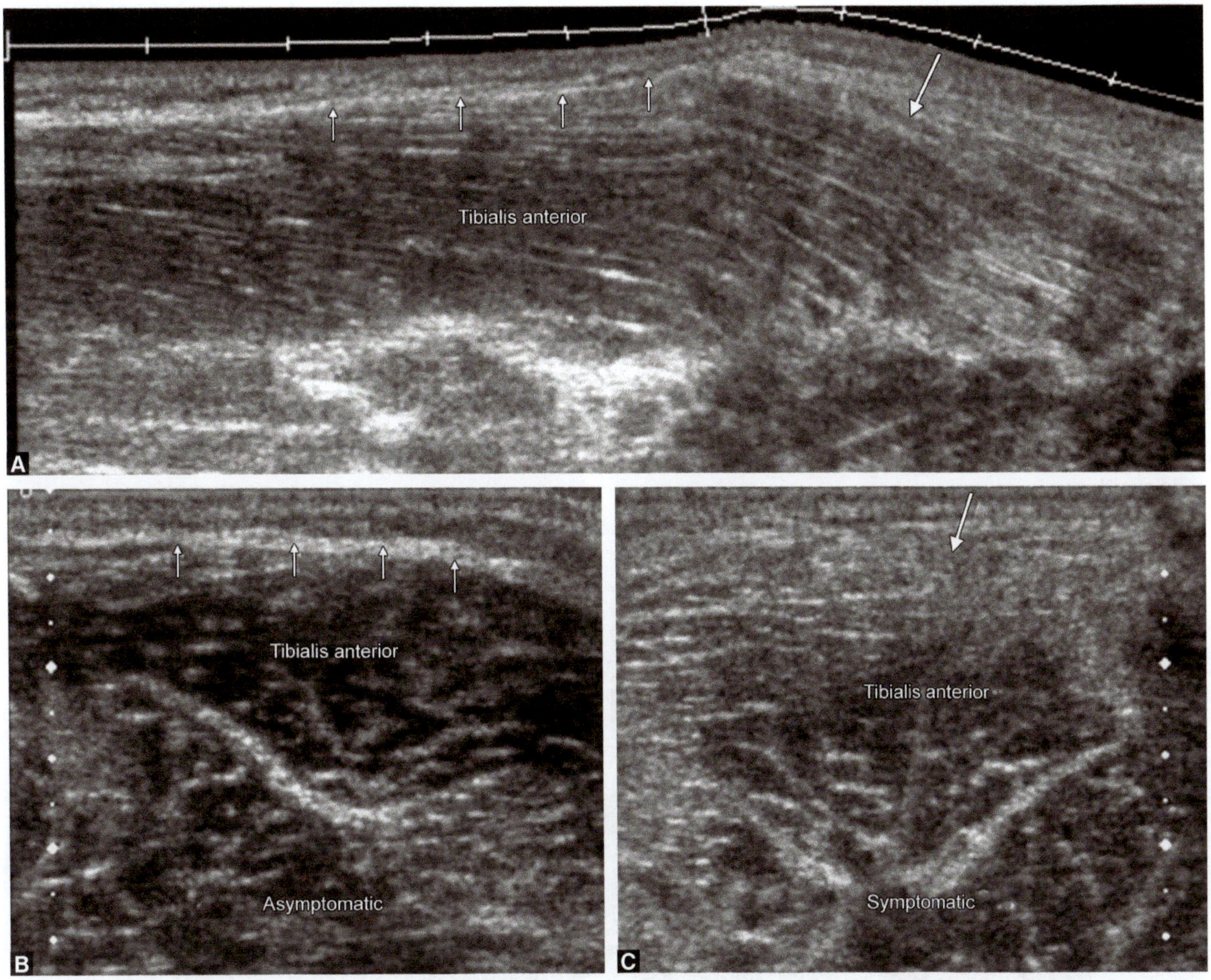

Figs. 2A to C: Long-axis (A) and transverse (B and C) images show deficiency of the deep muscular fascia (small arrows in Fig. B) resulting in herniation of the tibialis anterior muscle belly (big arrow in Fig. C) at this site.

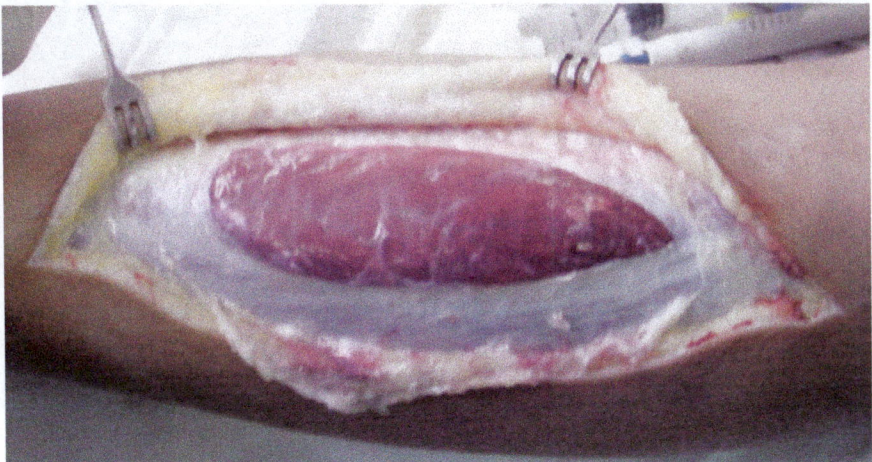

Fig. 3: Intraoperative appearance of the muscle hernia.

DIAGNOSIS

Transfascial herniation of the tibialis anterior muscle belly due to a defect in the deep fascia.

Case 69

Morel-Lavallée Lesion

■ CLINICAL HISTORY

A 26-year-old male presented with a progressively increasing swelling along lateral aspect of the thigh following a road traffic accident.

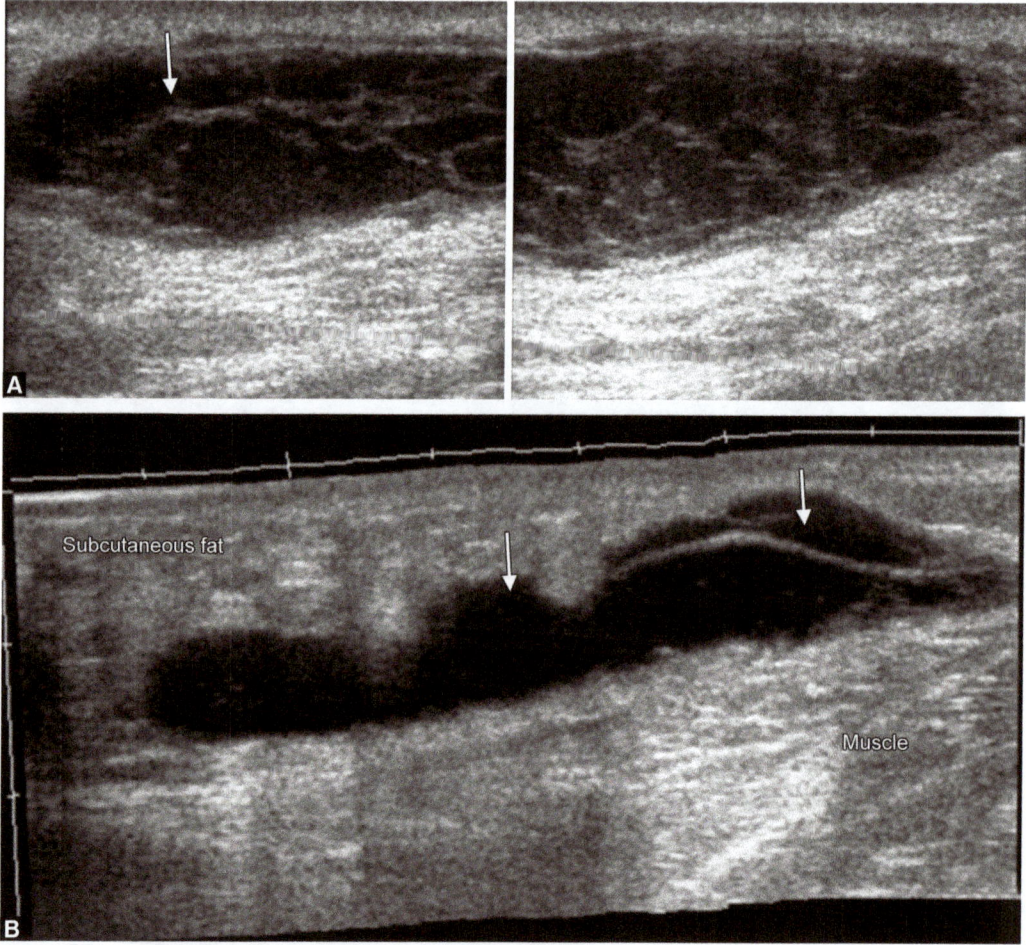

Figs. 1A and B: Long-axis images show a well-localized complex (arrows) collection between the subcutaneous fat and the muscle (A and B). Multiple low-level internal echoes are seen within the collection (arrow in A).

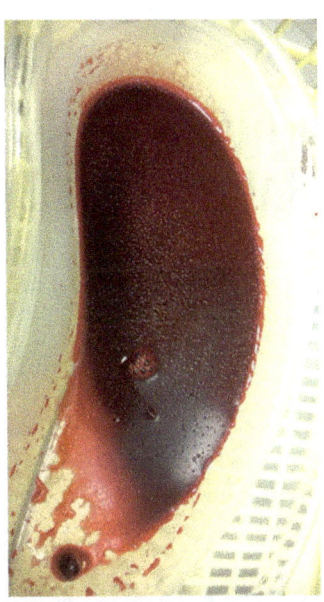

Fig. 2: Aspiration of the collection along the subcutaneous plane yielded blood.

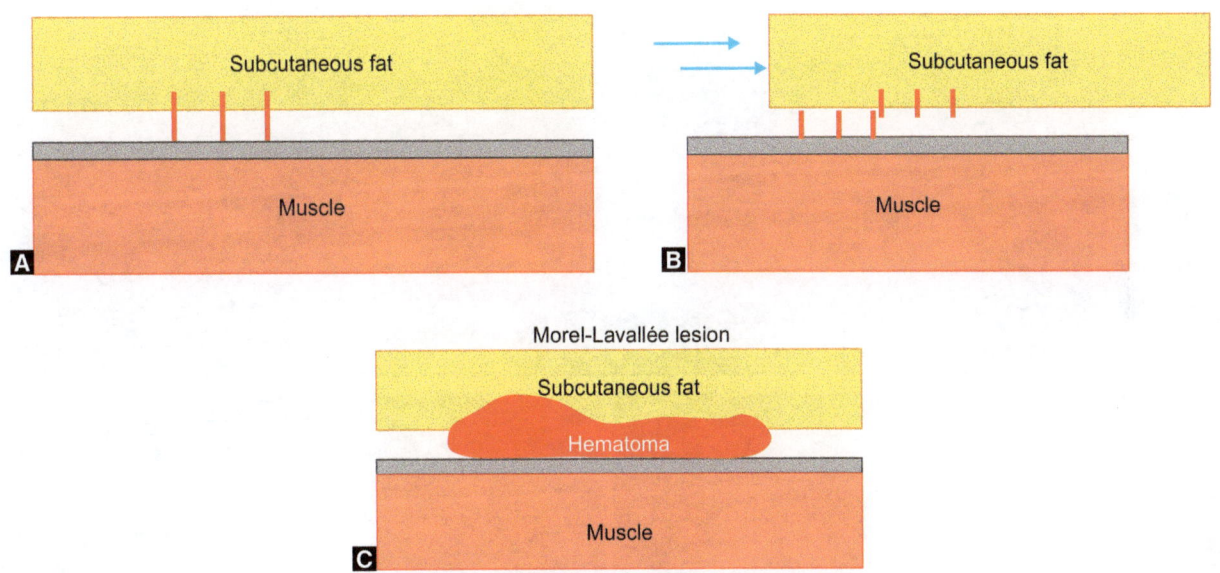

Figs. 3A to C: (A) Morel-Lavallée pathophysiology; (B) High-velocity forces cause shearing of the skin and subcutaneous fat over the deep fascia with disruption of perforating vessels and lymphatics; and (C) Discontinuity of the blood vessels results in formation of a hematoma between the subcutaneous fat and the deep fascia.

DIAGNOSIS

Chronic hematoma in the along the fascial plane between the subcutaneous fat and the muscle fascia (Morel-Lavallée lesion) (Figs. 1 and 2).

DISCUSSION

Morel-Lavallée lesions occur in the setting of a high velocity shearing injury, where an internal degloving injury occurs between the subcutaneous fat and the deep fascia. Rupture of the traversing vessels results in the formation of a hematoma (Figs. 3A to C).

CASE 70

Tendinosis of the Achilles Tendon with an Interstitial Tear

■ CLINICAL HISTORY

A 56-year-old man presented with chronic pain and fullness along the posterior aspect of the ankle since 2 months. He is known to have diabetes mellitus since 12 years.

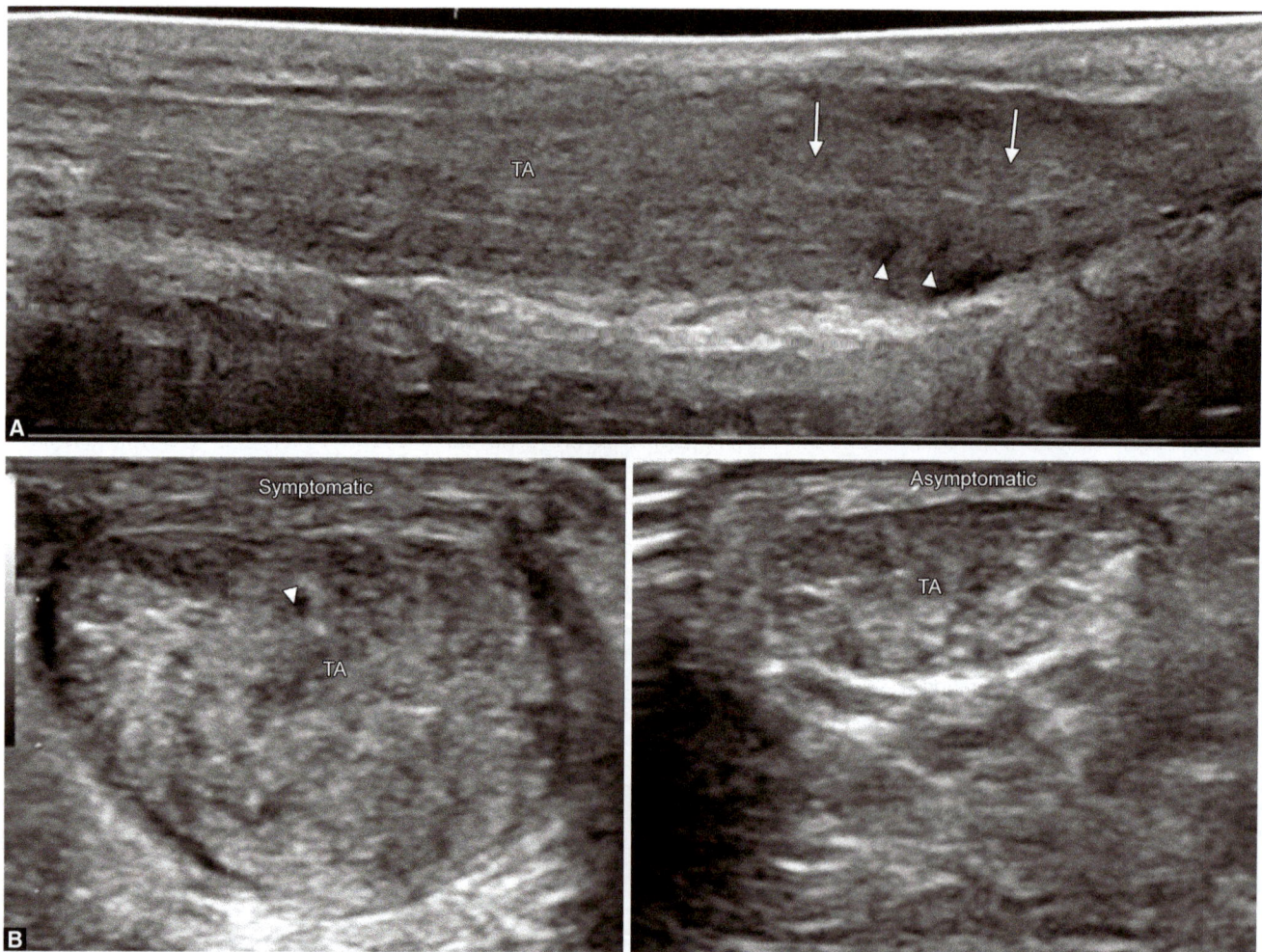

Figs. 1A and B: (A) The Achilles tendon (TA) appears diffusely thickened and hypoechoic (arrows). Few interstitial tears are seen within the tendon as anechoic clefts (arrowheads); and (B) On the short-axis image, the affected tendon appears rounded and globular in comparison with the asymptomatic tendon, which shows flattened appearance. The normal TA has a mildly flattened appearance wherein the transverse diameter of the tendon is more than that of the anteroposterior diameter.

DIAGNOSIS

Diffuse tendinosis of the Achilles tendon (TA) with a focal interstitial tear.

DISCUSSION

- The TA is formed by the aponeuroses of the medial and lateral gastrocnemius and the soleus muscles (triceps surae) in the middle third of the leg. Gastrocnemius muscle forms the larger volume of the TA.[1] The TA is devoid of a true tendon sheath and is instead covered by a fibrous layer known as paratenon. The paratenon is formed by two layers of thin fibrous tissue.[2] The primary function of paratenon is to provide nutrition to the AT through the internal mesotendal blood vessels and reduce friction during tendon movement.
- The TA measures 12–15 cm in length. Approximately 2–6 cm proximal to its calcaneal insertion, a zone of hypovascularity (critical zone) is identified within the TA where tendinosis and tears most often occur. Proximally, the tendon derives nutrition from the muscular branches of the gastrocnemius. The distal end of the TA is supplied by the periosteal vessels along the calcaneal insertion.
- As the TA courses caudally, there is a 90° turn in the fibers as a result of which the gastrocnemius fibers are located laterally and the soleus fibers are located medially at the calcaneal insertion of the TA.[3] A fibrocartilage is seen at the site of calcaneal attachment of the TA known as enthesis.
- The retrocalcaneal bursa is an anatomical bursa located at the site of TA insertion. Its primary function is to reduce friction between the posterior margin of the calcaneum and the TA. The retro-Achilles bursa is an adventitial bursa located between the TA and the subcutaneous tissues.
- Kager's fat is a triangular-shaped fat pad lying immediately anterior to the TA.
- *Spectrum of injuries to the TA* (Fig. 2):[1]
  - Tendinosis
  - Insertional tendinosis
  - Peritendinitis
  - Partial-thickness tear
  - Full-thickness tear.

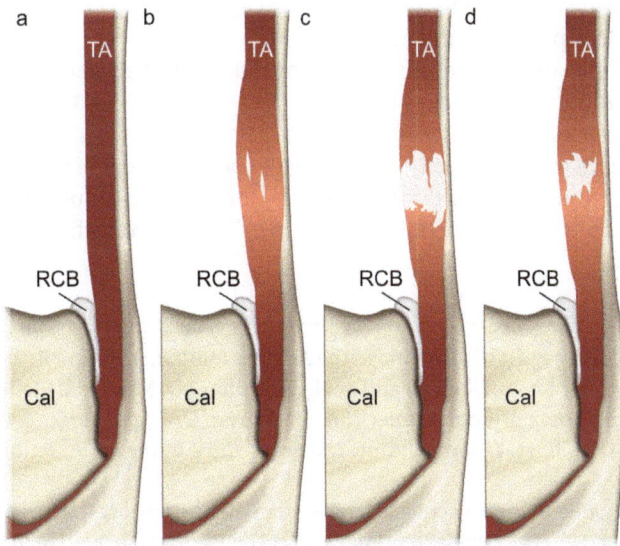

Fig. 2A: Spectrum of common pathologies affecting the Achilles tendon (TA). a: Normal Achilles tendon; b: Diffuse tendinosis with interstitial tears; c: Full-thickness tear of the Achilles tendon; and d: Partial-thickness tear of the Achilles tendon. (RCB: retrocalcaneal bursa; Cal: calcaneum)

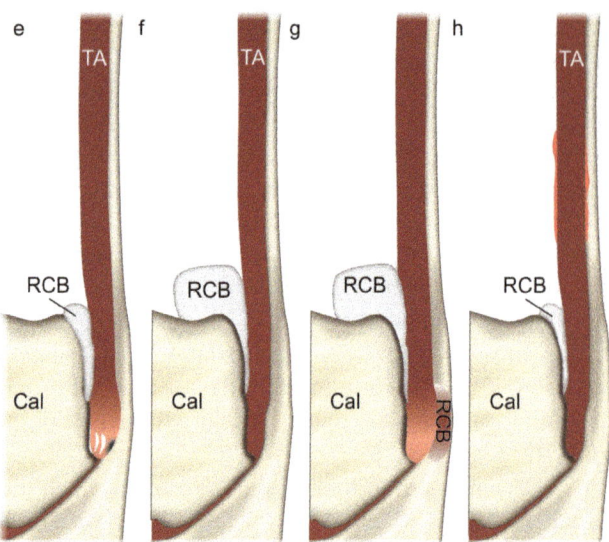

Fig. 2B: Spectrum of common pathologies affecting the Achilles tendon (TA). e: Insertional tendinosis with calcification; f: Retrocalcaneal bursitis; g: Haglund's syndrome [retrocalcaneal bursitis (RCB) + insertional tendinosis + retro-Achilles bursitis (RAB)]; and h: Paratenonitis. (Cal: calcaneum)

- *Role of ultrasound (US) in assessment of TA injuries*:
    - To confirm the presence of a tear
    - Differentiation of a partial thickness from a full-thickness tear
    - Identification of the location of tear
    - Assessment of distance between the apposing edges of a tear
    - Evaluation of adjacent structures, i.e. the plantaris tendon, retrocalcaneal bursa, and retro-Achilles bursa
    - Postoperative assessment of tendon healing.
- *Ultrasound characteristics of tendinosis involving the TA*:
    - Focal or diffuse thickening of the tendon resulting in fusiform enlargement (Figs. 1A and B). On the short axis, the TA appears more rounded compared to the normal oval appearance
    - Loss of echogenic fibrillary pattern of the native tendon
    - Intratendinous hypoechoic areas represent hypoxic or mucoid degeneration[4]
    - Intratendinous calcification
    - Thickening of the retrocalcaneal bursa is may be seen
    - Power Doppler shows increased vascularity within the involved segment of the tendon. Power Doppler examination of the TA should ideally done with plantar flexion of the foot so as to reduce the intratendinous pressure.[5]
- Peritendinitis is visualized on US as hypoechoic soft tissue or fluid surrounding the TA.

REFERENCES

1. Schweitzer ME, Karasick D. MR imaging of disorders of the Achilles tendon. AJR Am J Roentgenol. 2000;175:613-25.
2. Saltzman C, Bonor S. Tendon problems of the foot and ankle. In: Lutter LD, Mizel MS, Pfeffer GB (Eds). Orthopaedic Knowledge Update: Foot and Ankle, 1st edition. Rosemont: American Academy of Orthopaedic Surgeons; 1994. p. 270.
3. Root ML, Orien WP, Weed JH. Clinical Biomechanics: Normal and Abnormal Function of the Foot. Los Angeles: Clinical Biomechanics; 1977.
4. Bianchi S, Martinoli C. Ultrasound of the Musculoskeletal System. Berlin: Springer; 2007. pp. 817-23.
5. Zanetti M, Metzdorf A, Kundert HP, et al. Achilles tendons: clinical relevance of neovascularization diagnosed with power Doppler US. Radiology. 2003;227:556-70.

CASE 71

Chronic Partial-thickness Tear of the Achilles Tendon

■ CLINICAL HISTORY

A 62-year-old man presented with chronic pain along the posterior aspect of the ankle since 6 months. He has developed a limp since the past 3 weeks.

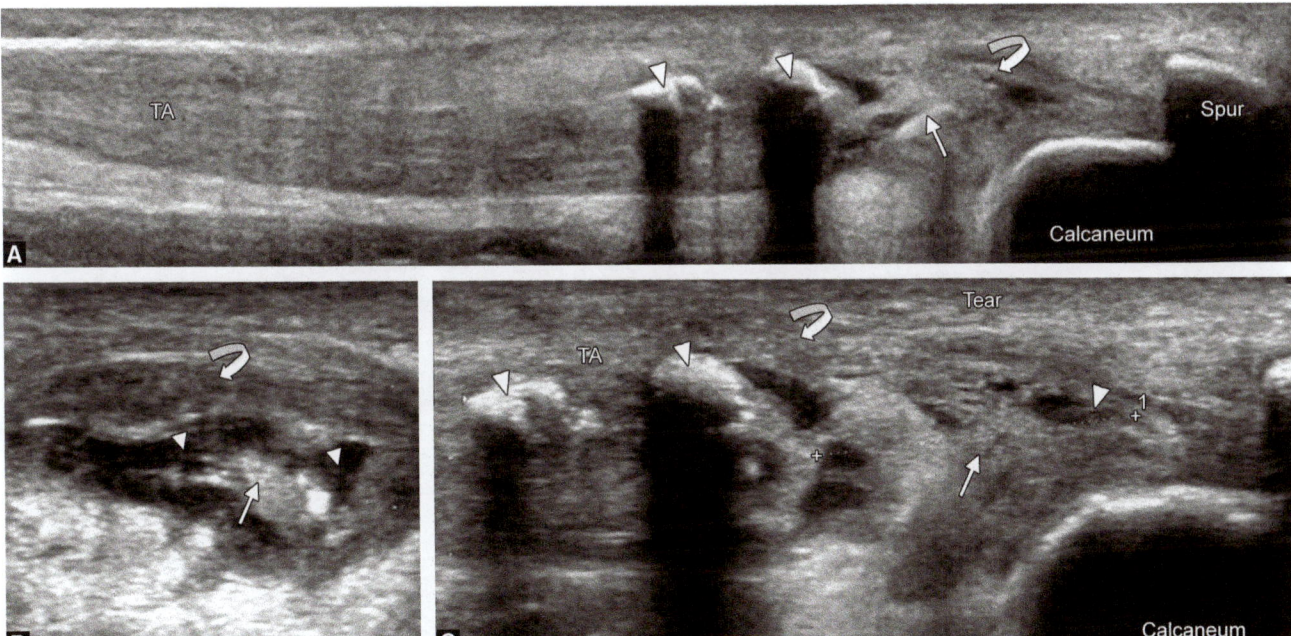

Figs. 1A to C: A high-grade partial-thickness tear (arrows) of the Achilles Tendon (TA) is seen in the ischemic zone. Few residual fibers (curved arrows) are seen bridging the tear. The torn edges appear hypoechoic and have calcifications (arrowheads). The involved segment of the tendon appears thickened and heterogeneous (B). Long-axis views (A and C) show enthesopathic changes (spur) at the calcaneal insertion of the TA.

■ DIAGNOSIS

Chronic partial-thickness tear of the Achilles tendon (TA).

■ DISCUSSION

- Achilles tendon tears may be either partial thickness or full thickness.
- Intratendinous hypoxia is the most common etiology identified in TA tears.[1]

- *Ultrasound (US) features in partial-thickness tear of the TA:*
    - Anechoic clefts within the TA (Figs. 1A to C). The clefts are generally oriented along the long-axis of the tendon fibers.
    - Thinning of the mid-portion of the tendon.
    - In the setting of tendinosis, a partial-thickness tear should be suspected if the anteroposterior diameter of the TA measures more than 1 cm and the anterior surface of the tendon appears irregular.[2]
    - Neovascularity on power Doppler along the margins of a chronic tear is indicative of a healing process.
- In a suspected TA tear, TA must be examined with the foot in maximum plantar and dorsiflexion positions. An occult tear may become more obvious on dorsiflexion.
- Ultrasound elastography has emerged as a promising tool in identifying the tendon stiffness and identifying areas of early tendon failure.

REFERENCES

1. Fox JM, Blazina ME, Jobe FW, et al. Degeneration and rupture of the Achilles tendon. Clin Orthop Relat Res. 1975;107:221-4.
2. Hartgerink P, Fessell DP, Jacobson JA, et al. Full-versus partial-thickness Achilles tendon tears: sonographic accuracy and characterization in 26 cases with surgical correlation. Radiology. 2001;220:406-12.

Case 72

Full-thickness Tear of Achilles Tendon

■ CLINICAL HISTORY

A 45-year-old man presented with a limp following a direct blunt blow directly along the posterior aspect of the ankle.

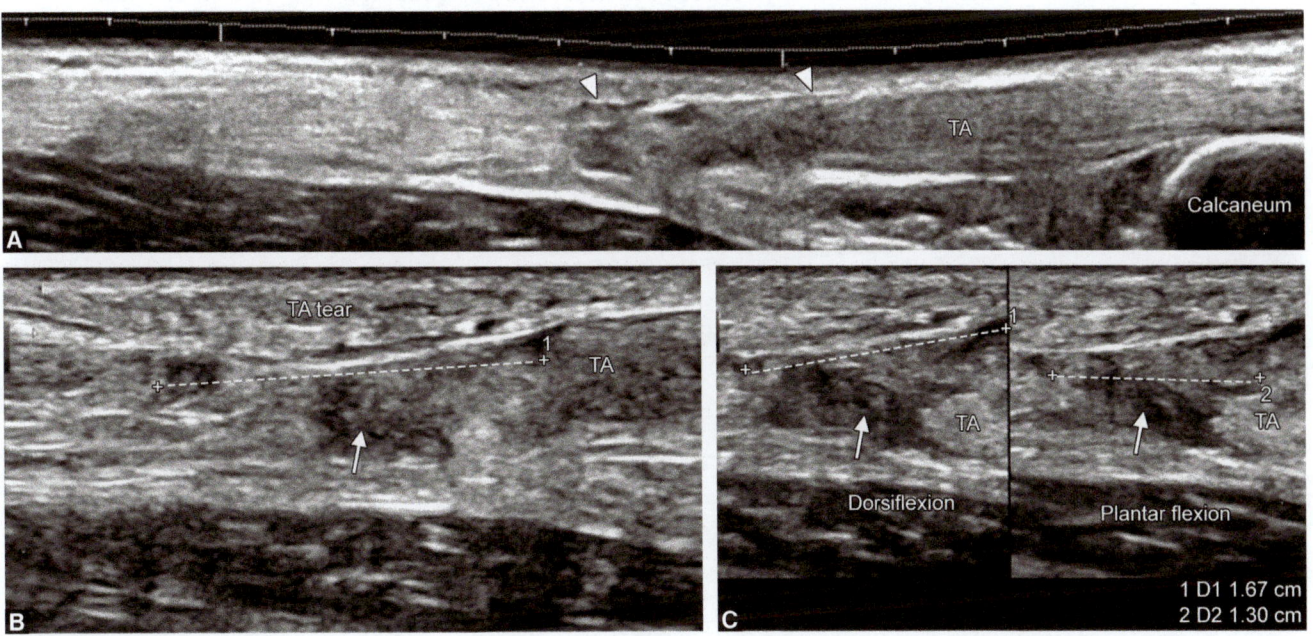

Figs. 1A to C: (A) Panoramic imaging in the long-axis shows a full-thickness tear (arrowheads) of the Achilles tendon (TA) is seen in the ischemic zone; and (B) Imaging of the tear with plantar flexion and dorsiflexion of the foot (C) shows movement at the margins of the tear (arrows).

■ DIAGNOSIS

Full-thickness tear of the Achilles tendon (TA).

■ DISCUSSION

- A full-thickness tear of the TA is seen on ultrasound (US) as complete discontinuity of the tendon along with retraction of the tendon stumps (Figs. 1A to C). The defect may be filled by an anechoic collection (hematoma) or echogenic Kager's fat.
- In chronic tears, the defect may be filled by hypoechoic soft tissue—which may represent either granulation tissue or fibrosis.

- *Reporting checklist for US evaluation of a TA tear:*
  - Full/partial-thickness tear
  - Size of the tear (craniocaudal)
  - Change in the tear size during plantar flexion and dorsiflexion of the foot
  - Distance between the lower margin of the tear and the calcaneal insertion of the TA
  - Herniation of Kager's fat between the torn ends (herniation of Kager's fat within the defect prevents approximation of the torn margins)
  - Condition of the torn margins, i.e. irregular margins, calcification, and hypoechoic appearance
  - Presence or absence of neovascularity (on power Doppler) along the torn margins
  - Look for atrophy in the gastrocnemius and soleus muscle bellies (muscle atrophy in a chronic tear is associated with a poor outcome following a tendon repair)
  - Fluid or synovial hypertrophy in the retrocalcaneal bursa
  - Integrity of the plantaris tendon
- The postoperative TA always appears thickened on US. Sutures are visualized as hyperechoic curvilinear structures embedded within the tendon.
- Serial US scans show gradual bridging of the defect with irregular soft tissue.
- Postoperative TA shows increased vascularity between 3 months and 6 months following which it declines.

Insertional Calcific Tendinosis of Achilles Tendon

CLINICAL HISTORY

A 44-year-old man who was an avid marathon runner, presented with pain along the posterior aspect of the heel since 5 months.

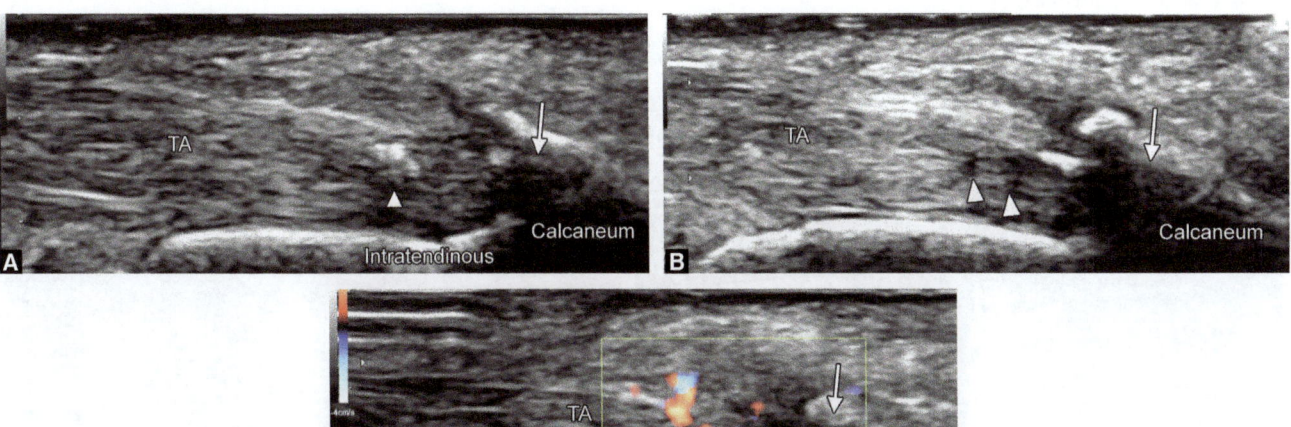

Figs. 1A to C: (A and B) Long-axis images show enthesopathic changes (arrows) are at the calcaneal attachment of the Achilles tendon (TA) along with intratendinous calcification (arrowhead) and interstitial tears (triangles) in the peri-insertional fibers; and (C) Power Doppler shows considerable intratendinous vascularity in the involved segment of the tendon.

DIAGNOSIS

Insertional calcific tendinosis of the Achilles tendon (TA).

DISCUSSION

- Insertional tendinosis of the TA is histologically characterized by microscopic tears, intratendinous calcification or ossification, and enthesopathic changes.
- Ultrasound (US) features of insertional tendinosis are similar to those of chronic tendinosis. Involvement of the retrocalcaneal fibers of the TA is the most characteristic feature.
- *Ultrasound findings in insertional tendinosis are*:
  - Hypoechogenicity and enlargement of the tendon
  - Interstitial tears
  - Intratendinous calcification at the site of enthesis (Figs. 1A to C)
  - Power Doppler shows increased vascularity during active inflammation.
- In refractory cases, platelet-rich plasma (PRP) injection may be done under US guidance at the site of inflammation. Alternatively, US-guided prolotherapy may also be performed.

CASE 74

Retrocalcaneal Bursitis

■ CLINICAL HISTORY

A 47-year-old woman presented with pain and tenderness along the posterior aspect of the ankle since 2 weeks. She is a known case of psoriasis.

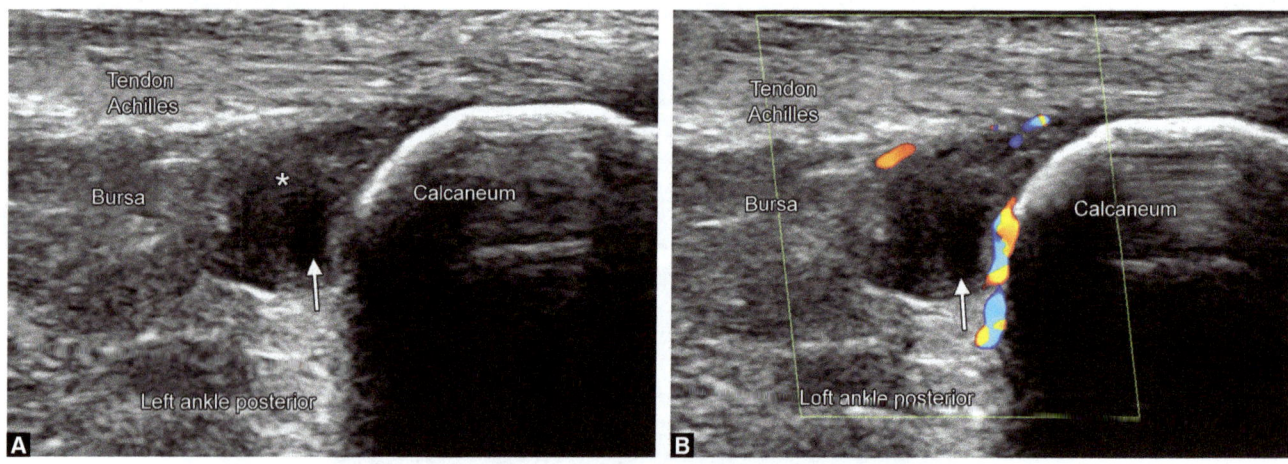

Figs. 1A and B: Long-axis images show enlargement of the retrocalcaneal bursa (arrows) along with synovial hypertrophy (*). Power Doppler (Fig. B) shows presence of vascularity.

■ DIAGNOSIS

Retrocalcaneal bursitis.

■ DISCUSSION

- Common causes of retrocalcaneal bursitis are Achilles tendinosis, inflammatory arthropathies, and overuse syndromes (e.g. runners).
- Retrocalcaneal bursa is considered abnormal when it measures more than 2 mm in the anteroposterior dimension and more than 6 mm in the craniocaudal dimension.[1]
- Ultrasound (US) may show synovial hypertrophy within the retrocalcaneal bursa. Presence of vascularity on power Doppler suggests active inflammation (Figs. 1A and B).
- Ultrasound-guided intrabursal injection of a combination of local anesthetic and a corticosteroid may be done in refractory cases.
- Haglund syndrome is a triad of retrocalcaneal bursitis, TA tendinosis, and retro-Achilles bursitis.

■ REFERENCE

1. Bottger BA, Schweitzer ME, El-Noueam KI, et al. MR imaging of the normal and abnormal retrocalcaneal bursae. AJR Am J Roentgenol. 1998;170:1239-41.

CASE 75

Haglund's Syndrome

CLINICAL HISTORY

A 62-year-old woman presented with painful swelling over the heel.

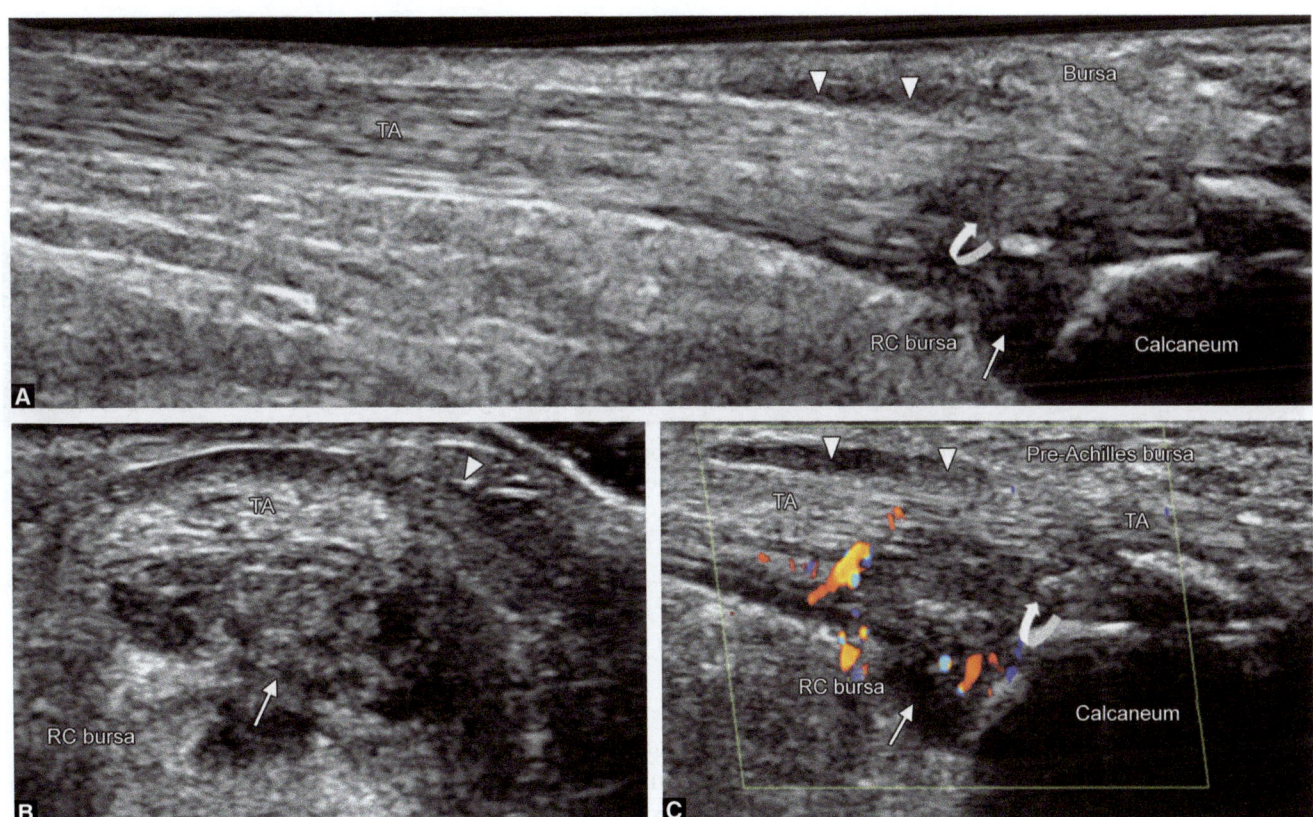

Figs. 1A to C: (A and B) Long-axis and short-axis images show thickening of the retrocalcaneal (straight arrows) and pre-Achilles (arrowheads) bursae. The distal segment of the Achilles tendon (TA) appears thickened and heterogeneous (curved arrows), suggestive of tendinosis; and (C) Color Doppler image shows vascularity within the thickened retrocalcaneal (RC) bursa and the involved segment of the TA.

DIAGNOSIS

Haglund's syndrome (retrocalcaneal bursitis along with insertional tendinosis of Achilles tendon and pre-Achilles bursitis).

Case 76

Tear of the Anterior Talofibular Ligament

■ CLINICAL HISTORY

A 23-year-old female encountered a twisting injury of the ankle 4 days ago while playing volleyball. She now presents with pain and swelling along the lateral aspect of the ankle.

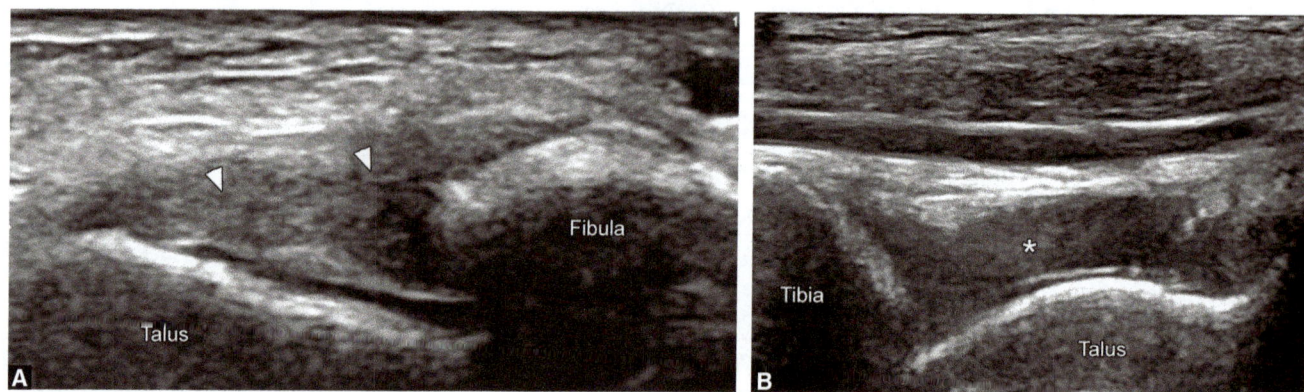

Figs. 1A and B: (A) The anterior talofibular ligament (ATFL) appears diffusely thickened and hypoechoic (arrowheads); and (B) Mild effusion (*) is seen in the anterior tibiotalar joint recess.

■ DIAGNOSIS

Tear of the anterior talofibular ligament (ATFL).

■ DISCUSSION

- Ankle is the most commonly injured joint in sports-related injuries.[1]
- Anterior talofibular ligament is the most frequently injured ligament in acute ankle injuries.[2] Recurrent inversion injury causes damage to the lateral ligamentous complex, resulting in ankle instability.
- The ATFL extends from the anterior margin of the lateral malleolus till the talar body (Fig. 3). The ligament may be injured either along its midsubstance or at the site of its osseous attachment (most commonly the fibular attachment).
- *Ultrasound (US) findings in ATFL ligament injury*:
  - Effusion in the anterior tibiotalar joint recess (Figs. 1A and B)
  - Normal appearing or thickened ligament (grade I sprain) (Fig. 2A)
  - Partial discontinuity of the ligament fibers (grade II sprain) (Fig. 2B)
  - Complete discontinuity of the ligament (grade III sprain) (Fig. 2C)
  - Hematoma at the site of the ligament
  - Osseous avulsion injury
  - Grade I and II injuries are managed conservatively.

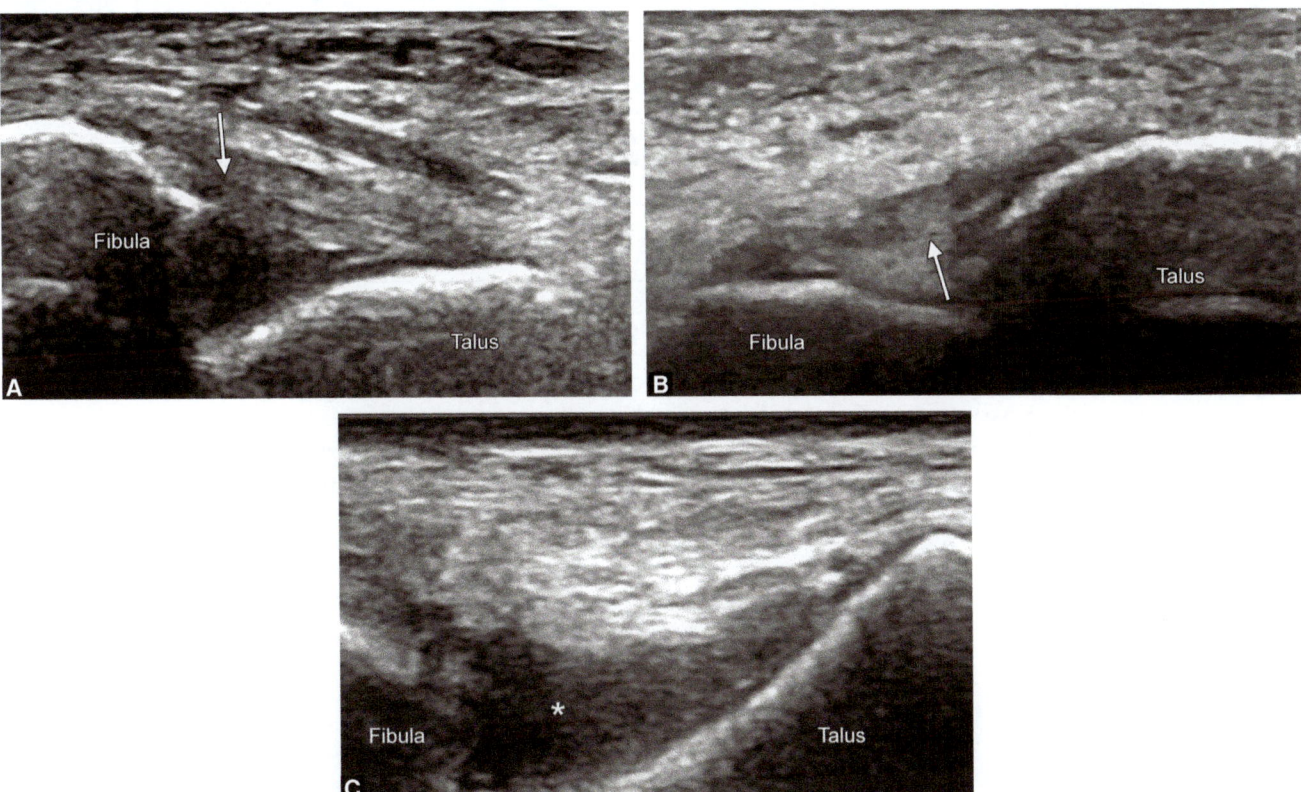

Figs. 2A to C: (A) Mild thickening (arrow) of the anterior talofibular ligament (ATFL); (B) Partial-thickness tear (arrow) of the ATFL; and (C) Nonvisualization of the ATFL (*) is suggestive of a complete tear. Mild effusion in the anterolateral gutter.

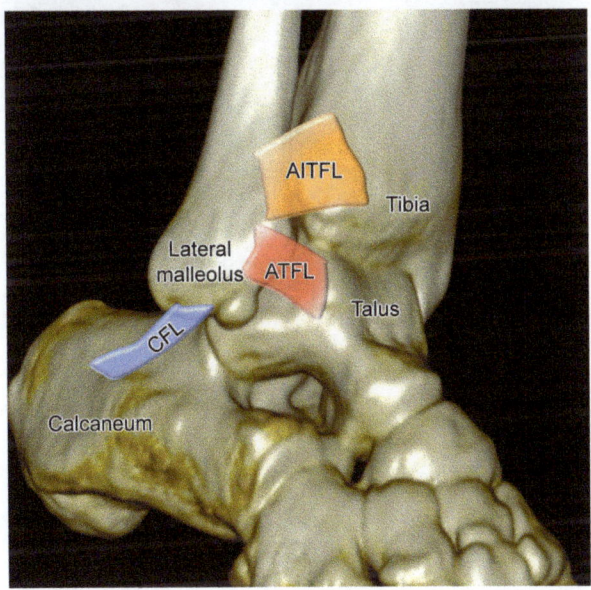

Fig. 3: Ligaments along the anterior and anterolateral aspect of the ankle.
(AITFL: anterior inferior tibiofibular ligament; ATFL: anterior talofibular ligament; CFL: calcaneofibular ligament)

■ REFERENCES

1. Garrick JG, Requa RK. The epidemiology of foot and ankle injuries in sports. Clin Sports Med. 1988;7:29-36.
2. Fong DT, Chan YY, Mok KM, et al. Understanding acute ankle ligamentous sprain injury in sports. Sports Med Arthrosc Rehabil Ther Technol. 2009;1:14.

Case 77

Chronic Tophaceous Gout

CLINICAL HISTORY

A 51-year-old male presented with a progressively increasing painless swelling over the lateral malleolus of the left ankle. He is known to have high serum uric acid levels.

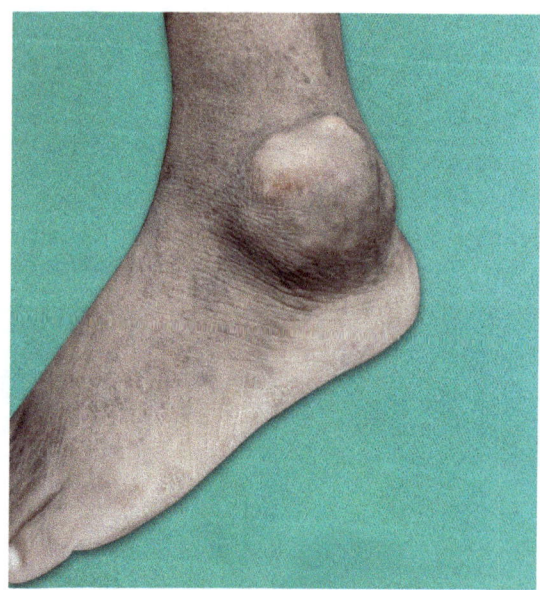

Fig. 1: Progressively increasing painless swelling over the lateral malleolus since 6 years.

Chronic Tophaceous Gout

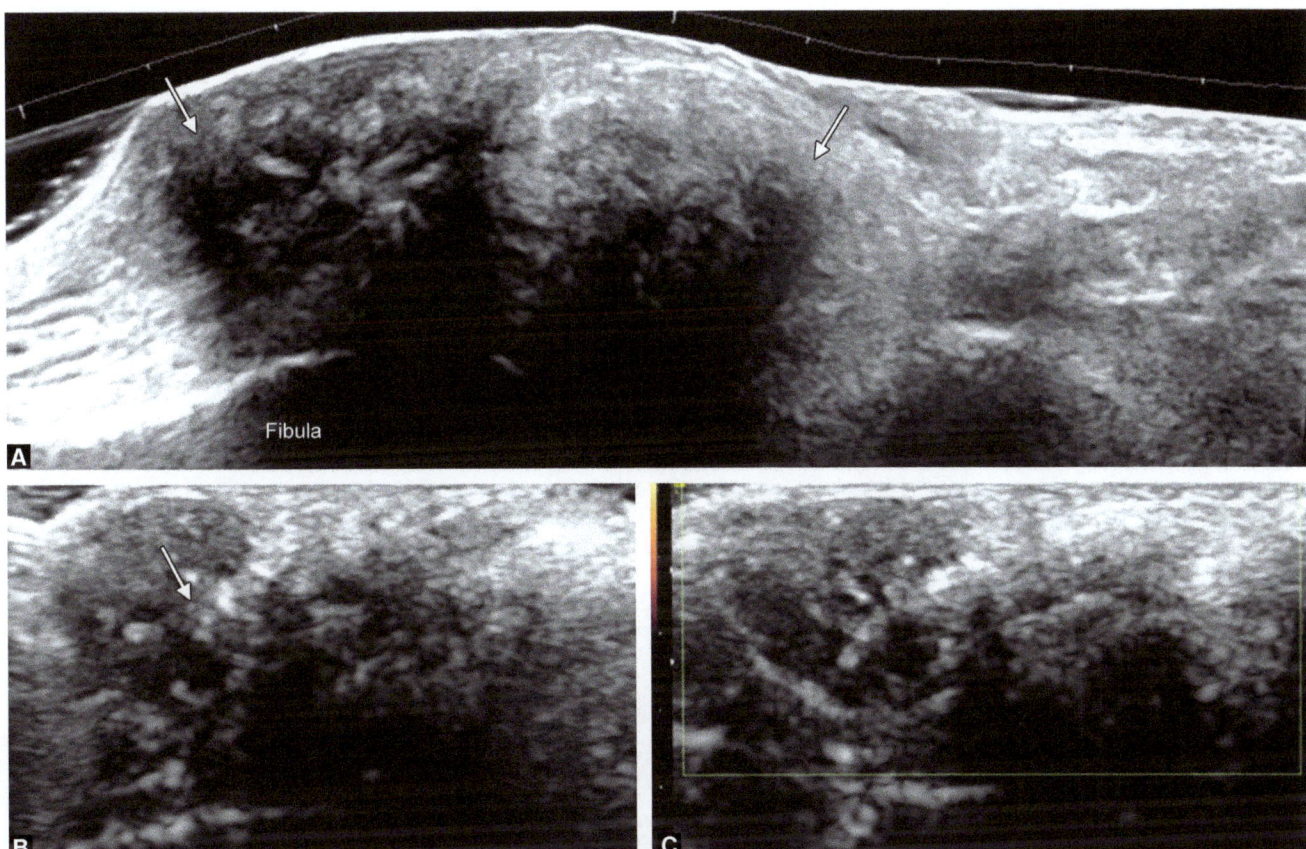

Figs. 2A to C: Long-axis (A) and transverse (B and C) images of the swelling over the lateral malleolus show diffuse soft tissue calcification (arrows) with distal shadowing over the lateral malleolus. Power Doppler does not show any significant intralesional vascularity.

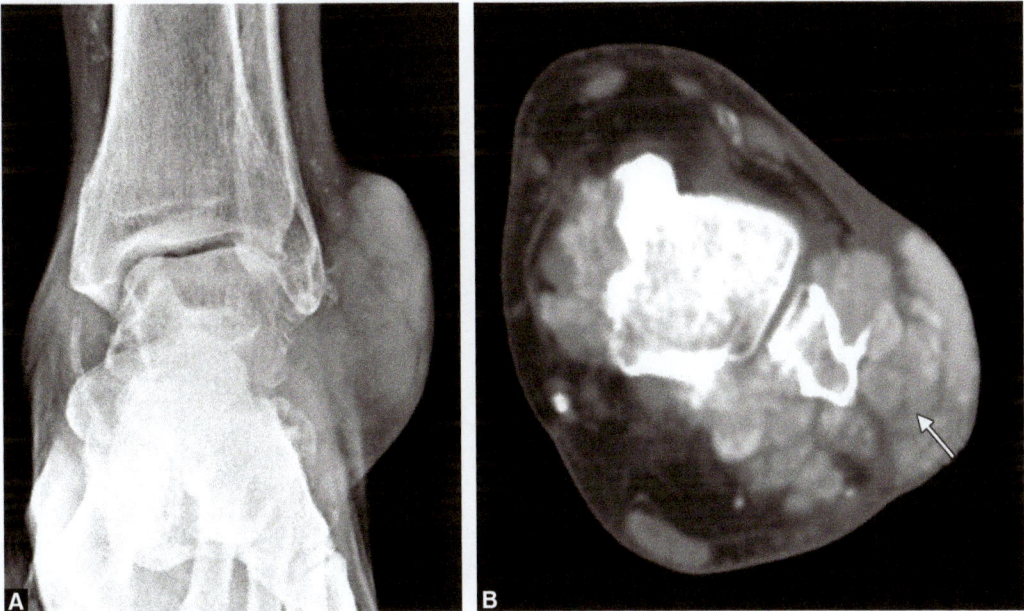

Figs. 3A and B: Frontal radiograph (A) and axial computed tomography (CT) image (B) show periarticular amorphous soft tissue calcification (arrow) along the lateral and posterior aspects of the ankle.

DIAGNOSIS

Chronic tophaceous gout.

DISCUSSION

- Chronic tophaceous gout is characterized by aggregates of uric acid crystals within the soft tissues of the body—predominantly in the periarticular regions (Figs. 1 and 3).
- The tophi appear as heterogeneously echogenic masses with hypoechoic areas interspersed (Figs. 2A to C). Distal shadowing and echogenicity of the nodules depend on the degree of calcification.
- Power Doppler does not show any intralesional vascularity.

Case 78

Interstitial Tear of the Tibialis Posterior Tendon with Tenosynovitis

■ CLINICAL HISTORY

A 66-year-old woman presented with acute pain along the medial aspect of the ankle.

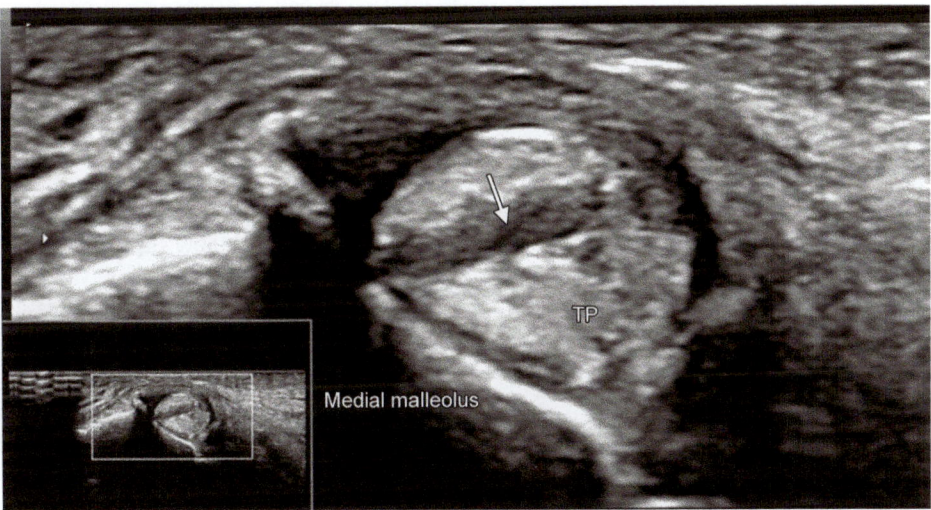

Fig. 1: A longitudinal tear (arrow) is seen in the retromalleolar segment of the tibialis posterior (TP) tendon. Anechoic fluid collection is seen within the tendon sheath.

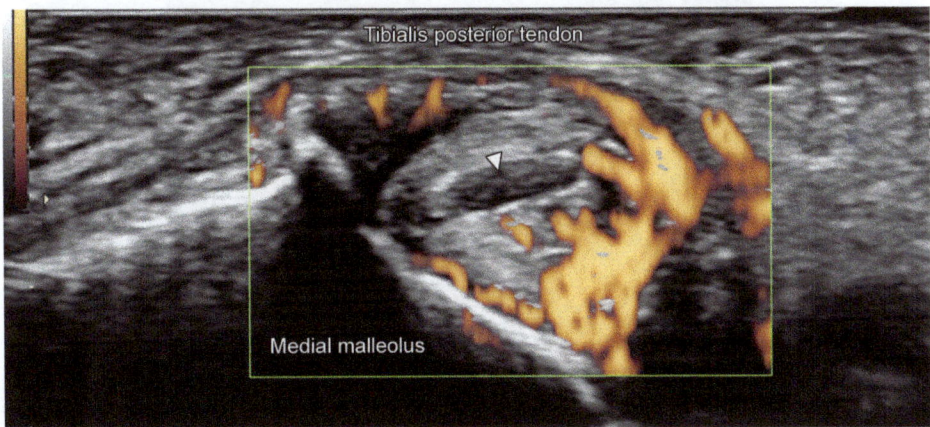

Fig. 2: Power Doppler shows considerable vascularity within the tibialis posterior (TP) tendon sheath and along the edges of the tear. Arrowhead points to the interstitial tear within the tendon.

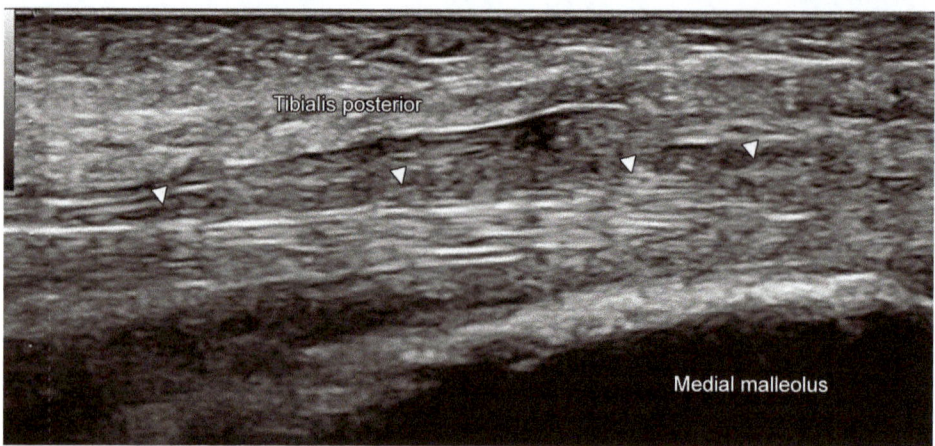

Fig. 3: A longitudinal tear (arrowheads) is seen in the retromalleolar segment of the tibialis posterior (TP) tendon.

■ DIAGNOSIS

Interstitial tear of the tibialis posterior (TP) tendon with tenosynovitis.

■ DISCUSSION

- The TP tendon is located posterior to the medial malleolus. It curves around the medial malleolus and runs anteriorly. A majority of the fibers of the TP tendon attach to the navicular bone (Fig. 4). Few slips of the tendon also attach to the three cuneiform bones and along the first, second, third, and fourth metatarsal bases.
- The supramalleolar and inframalleolar segments of the TP tendon have a synovial sheath which ends 1–2 cm proximal to its attachment at the navicular bone.

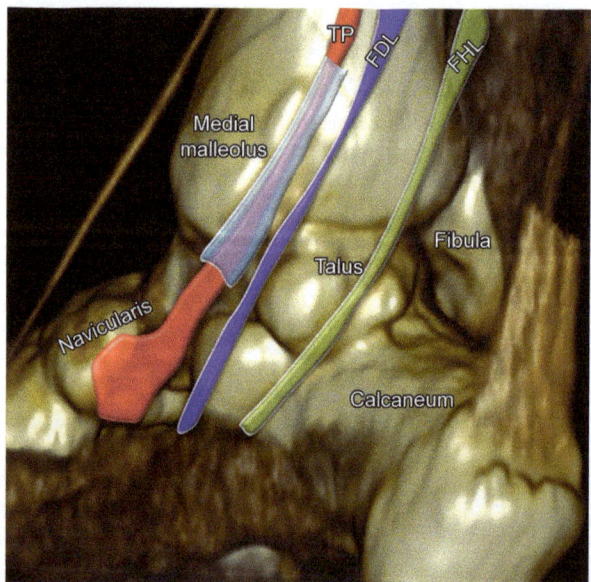

Fig. 4: Course and location of the tibialis posterior tendon along posteromedial aspect of the ankle. (FDL: flexor digitorum longus tendon; FHL: flexor hallucis longus tendon; TP: tibialis posterior tendon)

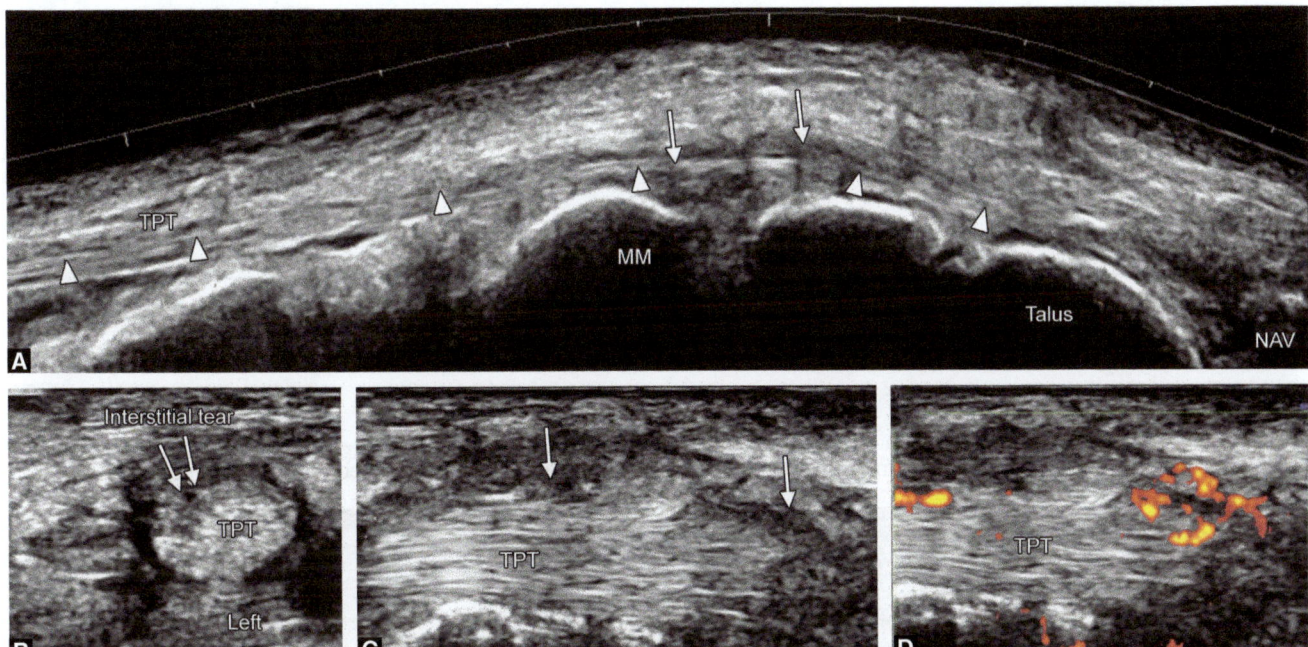

Figs. 5A to D: Long- and short-axis images show peritendinous soft tissue (arrows) along the inframalleolar segment of the tibialis posterior tendon (TPT) (arrowheads). Power Doppler image (D) shows marked vascularity within the peritendinous soft tissue. An interstitial tear (arrows) is seen at the periphery of the tendon (B). Long-axis image (A) shows presence of os navicularis (ON). (NAV: navicularis; MM: medial malleolus)

- Apart from being the main inverter of the foot, the TP tendon also causes its plantar flexion. The TP tendon also contributes to maintaining the medial longitudinal arch of the foot.
- Tibialis posterior tendon dysfunction may occur either due to tenosynovitis or tears of the TP tendon.
- Tibialis posterior tears most commonly occur at the level of the medial malleolus.
- Chronic tendinosis of the TP tendon results in interstitial tears and progressive flattening of the tendon ultimately leading to flatfoot. This condition is known as Tibalis posterior (TP) dysfunction.
- *Ultrasound (US) features of TP tear:*
  - Tendon thickening and intratendinous longitudinal split tears (Figs. 5A to D)
  - Elongated tendon with focal thinning
  - Complete discontinuity of fibers
  - Subacute and chronic tears show intratendinous vascularity on power Doppler images.
- Os navicularis, an accessory navicular bone close to the site of TP tendon insertion, can be visualized on US examination. Os navicularis is commonly implicated in tendinosis of the TP tendon.

Case 79

Interstitial Tear of Peroneus Brevis Tendon

■ CLINICAL HISTORY

A 41-year-old male presented with pain and mild swelling along the posterolateral aspect of the left ankle.

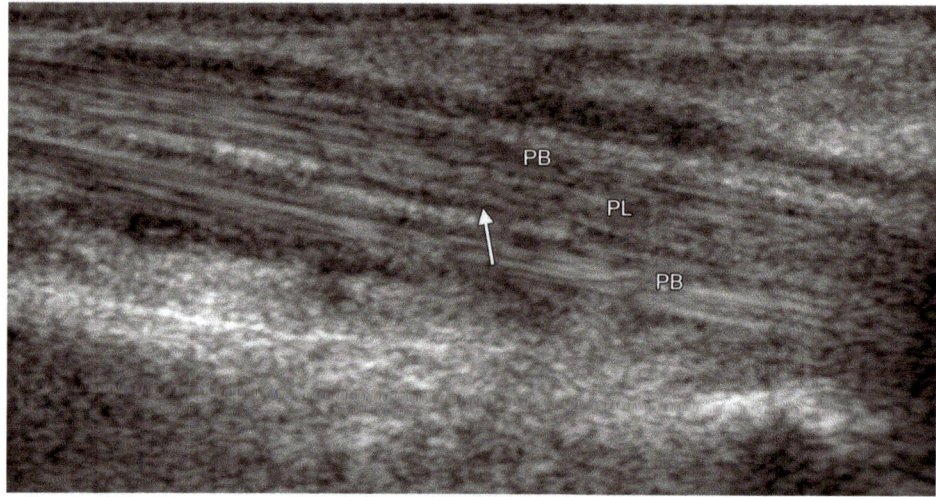

Fig. 1: The peroneus brevis (PB) tendon appears diffusely thickened. A longitudinal partial thickness tear is seen within the PB (arrow) splitting the tendon into two layers. The peroneus longus (PL) is seen interposed between the two layers of the PB tendon. Mild effusion is seen in the peroneal tendon sheath.

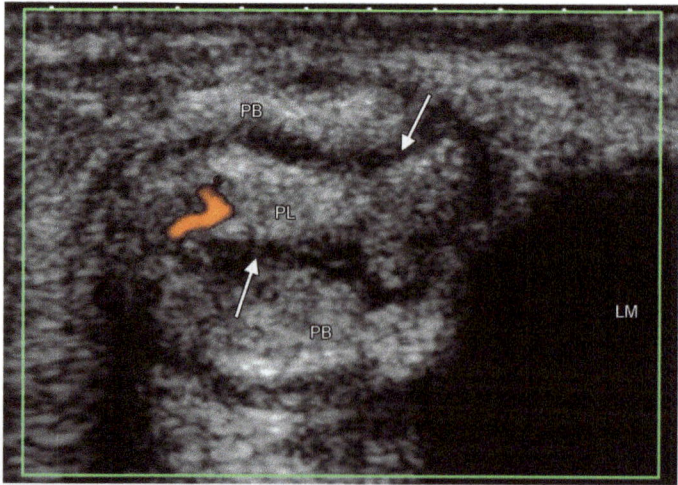

Fig. 2: Transverse image shows invagination of the peroneus brevis (PB) tendon by the peroneus longus (PL) tendon due to a defect in the PB caused by the vertical tear (arrows). Power Doppler shows mild vascularity within the torn PB tendon. (LM: lateral malleolus)

DIAGNOSIS

Interstitial tear of the peroneus brevis tendon with mild tenosynovitis involving the peroneal tendon sheath.

DISCUSSION

- The peroneus longus (PL) and PB are closely related tendons along the posterolateral aspect of the ankle and travel posterior and inferior to the lateral malleolus.
- The tendons are located in the retromalleolar groove along the posterior aspect of the fibula. The superior peroneal retinaculum passing above the tendons forms a fibro-osseous tunnel and holds the tendons in place and prevents bowstringing of the tendons (Fig. 3).

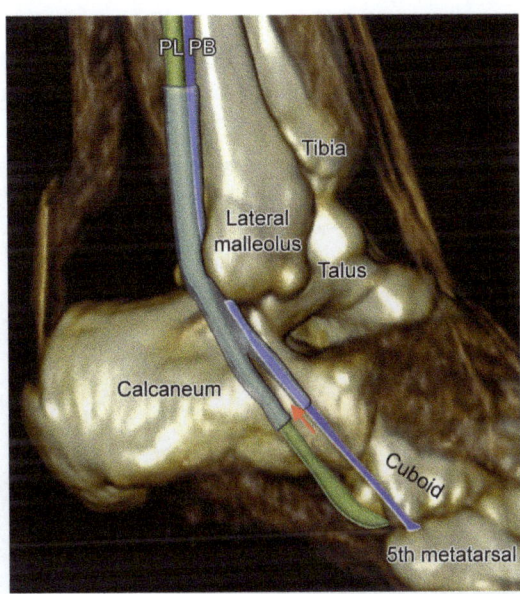

Fig. 3: Course and location of the peroneal tendons along posteromedial aspect of the ankle. [Peroneus longus (PL) tendon; peroneus brevis (PB) tendon; peroneal tubercle (red arrow)].

- Commonly seen peroneal tendon injuries include tenosynovitis, tendinosis, tears, and instability.
- Ultrasound (US) findings of peroneal tendon injuries are thickened and heterogeneous tendon morphology, split tears, and fluid in the tendon sheath. Split tears are more commonly seen in the PB tendon (Figs. 1 and 2). Tenosynovitis and tendinosis are commonly seen in inflammatory or infective conditions as well.
- Tears of the peroneal retinaculum may result in subluxation of the peroneal tendons from retromalleolar groove—demonstrated on the short-axis dynamic US images.

Case 80

Foreign Body Granuloma

■ CLINICAL HISTORY

A 33-year-old male with chronic pain along the plantar aspect of the foot since 4 months.

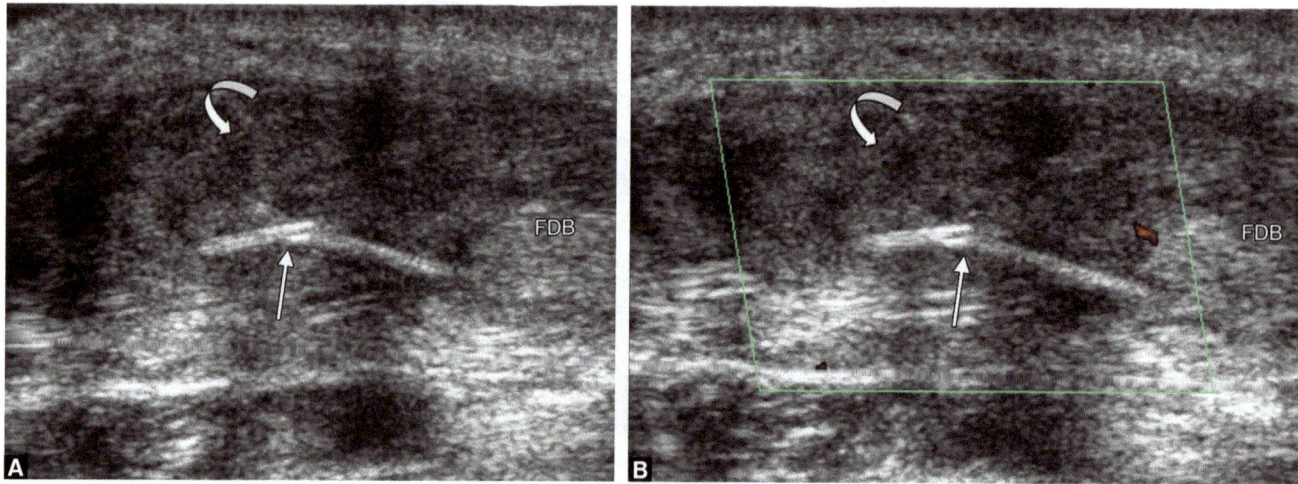

Figs. 1A and B: Two intramuscular foreign bodies (straight arrows) in the flexor digitorum brevis (FDB) muscle along the sole of the foot. Ill-defined soft tissue (curved arrows) is seen around the foreign bodies. Power Doppler does not show any significant vascularity in this soft tissue.

■ DIAGNOSIS

Foreign body (wooden splinter) granuloma within flexor digitorum brevis muscle belly.

■ DISCUSSION

- Ultrasound (US) is an excellent modality for detection and assessment of posttraumatic foreign bodies (FB). US can identify both radiodense and radiolucent FBs.
- On US, imaging features of FBs depend on the nature of the FB.
- A wooden FB would show posterior acoustic shadowing. Metal and glass FBs show posterior reverberations and comet-tail artifacts.
- On US, the FB granuloma is seen as a hypoechoic (Figs. 1A and B) halo surrounding the FB.
- It would be ideal to review the radiographs of the involved limb before scanning the area to identify the FB.
- In a preoperative scan, surface skin marking can be done to show the exact location of the FB. The distance between the skin surface and the FB should also be measured.

Case 81

Pyomyositis

CLINICAL HISTORY

A 62-year-old male presented with fever, leukocytosis, and a painful swelling along the plantar aspect of foot close to the lateral margin since 1 week.

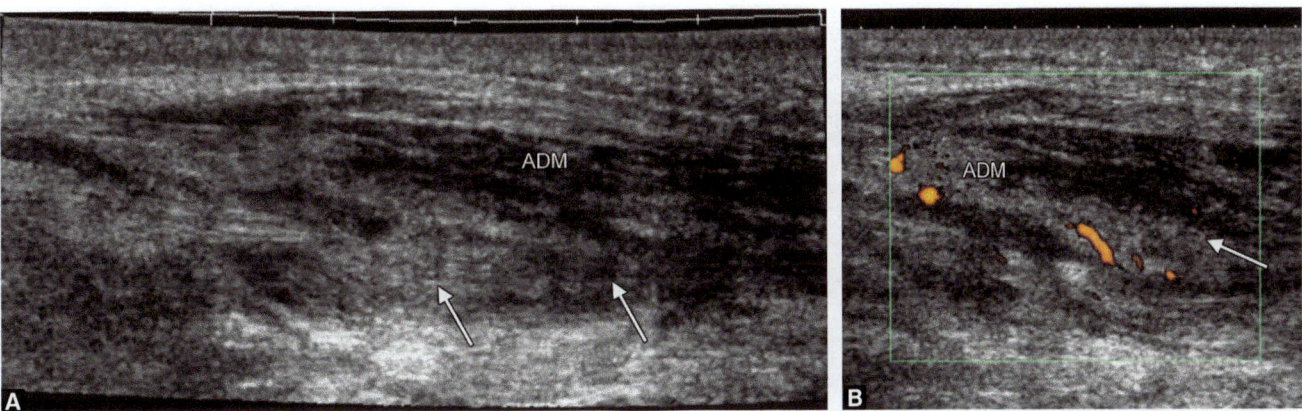

Figs. 1A and B: (A) The abductor digiti minimi (ADM) muscle appears heterogeneous and diffusely edematous (arrows) with loss of the normal pennate pattern. (B) Power Doppler shows mild vascularity (arrow) within the involved muscle.

DIAGNOSIS

Pyomyositis involving the abductor digiti minimi muscle belly.

DISCUSSION

- Pyomyositis commonly involves the muscles of the lower limb.
- It is commonly seen in patients having an immunocompromised status [e.g. human immunodeficiency virus (HIV)-acquired immunodeficiency syndrome (AIDS) and diabetes mellitus].
- *Ultrasound (US) features of pyomyositis*:
  - Muscle enlargement
  - Hyperechoic appearance of the muscle with increased vascularity (Figs. 1A and B)
  - Hypoechoic areas within the involved muscle belly suggest central necrosis and abscess formation.
- Ultrasound-guided aspiration of the collection may be done.

CASE 82

Plantar Fasciitis

CLINICAL HISTORY

A 57-year-old female presented with pain along the plantar aspect of the heel since 3 weeks.

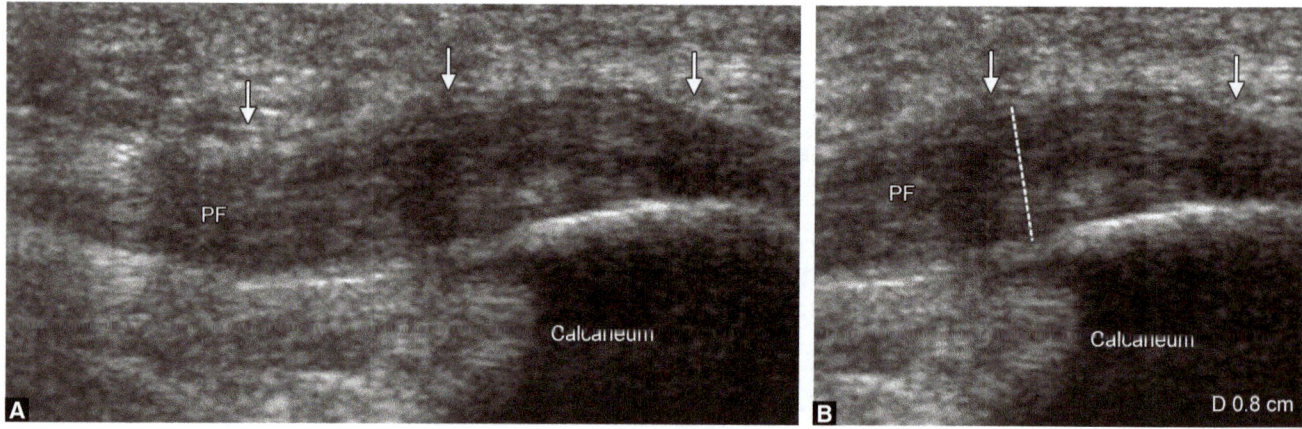

Figs. 1A and B: (A) The plantar fascia (PF) appears diffusely thickened and hypoechoic (arrows) on long-axis image; and (B) It measures 0.8 cm in thickness.

DIAGNOSIS

Plantar fasciitis.

DISCUSSION

- The plantar fascia predominantly originates from the medial calcaneal tuberosity. It is a fibrous aponeurosis that plays an important role in maintaining the medial longitudinal arch of the foot and distribution of forces and stresses of the foot during gait. The fascia consists of three cords—central, lateral and medial. The central cord is most commonly involved.
- *Common pathologies of the plantar fascia include:*
  - Plantar fasciitis
  - Rupture of plantar fascia
  - Plantar fibromatosis.
- Recurrent microtrauma to the plantar fascia results in microtears within the fascia, resulting in chronic low-grade inflammation, i.e. plantar fasciitis.

- Acute tears of the plantar fascia are relatively uncommon.
- Plantar fasciitis is commonly seen in marathon runners, sprinters, and people with obesity.
- *Ultrasound (US) features of plantar fasciitis*:
    - Thickened and hypoechoic appearance of plantar fascia (Figs. 1A and B)
    - Plantar fascia thickness more than 4.5–5 mm is considered abnormal. Alternatively, plantar fascia thickness by more than 1 mm when compared with the asymptomatic side
    - Edema in the adjacent plantar fascia
    - Increased vascularity on power Doppler images
    - Discontinuity of the fibers suggest microtears
    - Calcification within the plantar fascia.

Index

Page numbers followed by *f* refer to figure.

A

Abductor digiti minimi muscle 65, 165*f*
Abductor pollicis longus 74*f*, 76, 76*f*
Achilles tendinosis 152
Achilles tendon 144*f*-146*f*, 147, 149*f*
    calcaneal attachment of 151*f*
    chronic partial-thickness tear of 147
    distal segment of 153*f*
    full-thickness tear of 145*f*, 149
    high-grade partial-thickness tear of 147*f*
    insertional tendinosis of 151, 153
    normal 145*f*
    partial-thickness tear of 145*f*
    tendinosis of 144, 145
Acquired immunodeficiency syndrome 165
Acromioclavicular joint 16, 32*f*, 33*f*
    dislocation 32, 33
Acromioclavicular ligament, disruption of 33*f*
Adductor brevis 107*f*
    muscle bellies 106*f*
Adductor longus 106*f*
    muscle 107*f*
Adductor magnus 106*f*
    muscle 107*f*
Adductor muscles
    acute partial thickness tear of 106
    partial-thickness acute tear of 107
Amyloidosis 84
Anabolic steroid abuse 55
Anechoic clefts 148
Anechoic fluid 27*f*
    collection 159*f*
    mild 5*f*
Anechoic intrabursal fluid 121
Anisotropy 46*f*
Ankle 154
    anterior aspect of 155*f*
    anterolateral aspect of 155*f*
    lateral and posterior aspects of 157*f*
    medial aspect of 159
    posterior aspect of 144, 147, 149, 152
    posteromedial aspect of 160*f*, 163*f*
Ankylosing spondylitis 78
Arch, coracoacromial 2*f*
Arm
    abduction of 10
    overhead abduction of 29
    posterior aspect of 41
Arthropathy, inflammatory 90, 91, 152

B

Baker's cyst 135, 135*f*, 136, 137
    complications of 136
    contents of 136
    distal edge of 135*f*
    idiopathic 136
Biceps
    brachii muscle 20
    femoris 114, 136*f*
        tendon 114*f*
    long head of 1*f*, 8*f*, 15*f*, 20, 22*f*, 23*f*, 25*f*, 27*f*
    muscle, long-axis of 20*f*
    senosynovitis of long head of 16
    tear of long head of 20
    tendon 21*f*, 22*f*, 59*f*
        distal 46*f*, 59, 59*f*
        long head of 24*f*
        long-axis of 22*f*
        proximal fibers of 22*f*
        sheath 15*f*, 23*f*, 24, 74
Bicipital groove, level of 24*f*, 27*f*
Bicipitoradial bursitis 46, 46*f*, 47
Blood cell count 118
Bursal contents, evaluation of 121
Bursal surface tear 6, 6*f*
    partial-thickness 5*f*
Bursitis, chronic 121

C

Calcaneofibular ligament 155*f*
Calcific tendinosis 12, 51
Calcification
    hyperechoic zone of 61*f*
    intratendinous 111, 112*f*, 151, 151*f*
    migration of 13
Calcium 14*f*
    extrusion of 12
    periarticular 87*f*
    pyrophosphate dihydrate 87
Calf
    muscle injuries, assessment of 139
    posterior aspect of 138
Capsulitis, adhesive 26
Carpal bone 65*f*, 66*f*
Carpal tunnel syndrome 65
Cartilage
    articular 7*f*
    cap thickness 125
Chalk-like consistency 12
Chikungunya viral infection 46
Complex cyst 81*f*
Connective tissue 84
Contusion injuries 38
Coracohumeral ligament, normal 26*f*
Corticosteroids, intrabursal injection of 121
Crush injury over arm 36
Crystal deposition disease 86, 120*f*
Cuff tear 4
    retraction, stages of 9*f*
Cyst, paralabral 29, 30, 30*f*
Cysticercosis 42
    intramuscular 42

D

De Quervain's tenosynovitis 74, 76
Deep fibers, inflammation of 126*f*
Deep muscular fascia, deficiency of 141*f*
Deep venous thrombosis 139
Deltoid muscle 1*f*, 4*f*, 5*f*, 7*f*, 8*f*, 10*f*, 11*f*, 22, 25*f*, 27*f*
Diabetes mellitus 4, 110, 144, 165
Distal arm, anteromedial aspect of 36*f*
Distal biceps tendon, full-thickness tear of 59
Distal femoral shaft, anterior cortex of 124*f*
Distal phalanx 97*f*, 101*f*, 103*f*
Distal radius, dorsal cortex of 77*f*
Dorsal cortex, scalloping of 101*f*
Dorsal radial cortex 76*f*

E

Ecchymosis 104*f*, 106*f*, 113*f*, 138, 138*f*
Echogenic nodules, multiple 16*f*

Edema 115, 167
    periarticular 87
    peribursal 14*f*
Elbow 51*f*, 55*f*, 57*f*, 61*f*
    acute repetitive overstretching of 60
    anterior aspect of 46
    chronic repetitive overstretching of 60
    joint
        posterior aspect of 57*f*
        posterior dislocation of 60
    medial
        aspect of 51, 61*f*
        joint space of 60*f*
    pain, lateral 50
Empty bicipital groove 20*f*, 21*f*
Epicondylitis
    lateral 50
    medial 52
Epidermal inclusion cyst 81, 82
Erosions 91, 93
Erythematous painful swelling, acute 86
Erythematous tender swelling 86*f*
Exostosis 125
    smooth cortex of 125*f*
Extensor carpi
    radialis brevis 49
    ulnaris 49, 79*f*
Extensor compartment, tendon sheath of 76, 79
Extensor digitorum communis 49
Extensor origin, common 40, 49*f*
Extensor pollicis
    brevis 74*f*, 75*f*, 76
        tendon 76*f*
    longus tendon 97*f*
        full-thickness tear of 97
        traumatic full-thickness tear of 97
Extensor tendon 99*f*
    attritional tear of 77

F

Fascial plane 143
Fat
    lobules 34*f*
    necrosis, traumatic 34, 35
Fever 118, 165
Fibers
    discontinuity of 36*f*, 60, 167
    peri-insertional 151*f*
Finger
    dorsal aspect of 81*f*
    extensor tendon of 99
    flexor-tendon sheath of 98
    volar aspect of 88, 94*f*, 96*f*
First metacarpophalangeal joint, volar aspect of 86*f*

Flexor carpi radialis 63*f*
Flexor digitorum
    brevis muscle 164, 164*f*
    longus tendon 160*f*
    profundus 83*f*, 84*f*, 89*f*, 94*f*, 95*f*
    profundus tendon 96*f*
        full-thickness tear of 96
        traumatic full-thickness tear of 96
    superficialis 52*f*, 83*f*, 89*f*, 95*f*
        muscles 52
        tendon 84*f*, 94*f*, 96*f*
Flexor hallucis longus tendon 160*f*
Flexor origin, common 51, 52, 60*f*
Flexor pollicis longus 85*f*, 87*f*
Flexor tendons 65*f*, 66*f*, 73*f*, 88*f*, 98*f*
    of middle finger, tenosynovitis of 95
    sheath 73*f*, 94*f*, 95*f*
    tendinosis of 94
Foot
    dorsiflexion of 149*f*, 150
    necrosis, traumatic 35
    plantar aspect of 164, 165
Forearm, extensor aspect of 53*f*
Fracture
    morphology of 40*f*
    of humeral shaft, internal fixation of 39
Frozen shoulder 26
Full-thickness tear 5*f*-8*f*, 9, 18*f*, 21, 59*f*, 60*f*, 96*f*, 97*f*, 111, 130*f*, 145, 149*f*
Fusiform hypoechoic area, peri-insertional 127

G

Ganglion 29*f*, 64, 64*f*, 88
    cyst 88*f*
    paralabral 30
    ulnar aspect of 64*f*
Gastrocnemius
    head
        lateral 136*f*
        medial 136*f*-139*f*
    semimembranosus bursa 136, 136*f*, 137*f*
Giant-cell tumor 98-100
Glenohumeral joint capsule, normal appearance of 26*f*
Glenoid labrum 29*f*
Glomus
    bodies 102
    tumor 102, 103, 103*f*
Gluteus medius 111*f*
    deep and anterior fibers of 111
    tendon 110*f*
        partial-thickness tear of 110, 111
Gluteus minimus 111*f*, 112*f*
    tendon 112*f*

Gluteus tendinopathy 111
Gluteus tendons 111*f*
Granuloma, foreign body 164
Greater trochanter 108*f*, 110*f*, 111, 111*f*, 112*f*
Greater trochanteric
    bursa 108, 108*f*, 109, 111*f*, 112*f*
    pain syndrome 109
Greater tuberosity 10*f*, 1*f*, 2, 2*f*, 4*f*-7*f*, 11*f*, 12*f*, 22, 24*f*
    cortical irregularity over 6

H

Haglund's syndrome 146*f*, 152, 153
Hamate-trapezium level 67
Hamstring injuries 115
Hamstring tendons, high-grade tear of 114
Hansen disease 43
Heel, plantar aspect of 166
Hematoma 59*f*, 105, 106*f*, 107, 116, 117, 139*f*, 154
    chronic 143
    large 114*f*
Hemorrhage 136
Hemorrhagic bursa 121
Hemorrhagic superficial infrapatellar bursitis 123
Hip 118*f*
Human immunodeficiency virus 165
Humerus 25*f*
    posterior aspect of 55*f*
Hydroxyapatite crystal deposition 87
Hyperemia 61*f*, 87
Hypoechoic
    appearance 111
    areas 165
    rim, peripheral 61*f*
    solid lesion 53*f*, 71*f*, 72, 72*f*
Hypothyroidism 84
Hypoxia, intratendinous 147

I

Infraspinatus muscle, atrophy of 31
Injuries
    chronic 115
    penetrating 38, 96
Interosseous nerve, posterior 50
Interphalangeal joint, dorsal recess of 92*f*
Interstitial tear, focal 145
Intralesional vascularity, presence of 54
Intratendinous subscapularis calcification, extrusion of 14*f*
Ipsilateral knee, arthroplasty of 132

J

Joint
    capsule
        displace 118*f*
        inferior 26*f*
    effusion 90*f*
    glenohumeral 23*f*, 26*f*
    metacarpophalangeal 83*f*, 85*f*, 90, 105
Jumper's knee 126, 127

K

Kager's fat 145, 149
    herniation of 150
Knee 124*f*
    anterior aspect of 119, 120*f*, 130
    aspiration of 133
    extension, loss of 130
    extensor mechanism of 131
    pain, anterior 126
    posteromedial aspect of 135, 137
Knife injury 97

L

Labrum, posterior aspect of 29*f*
Leprosy 43
    three broad forms of 43
Lesser tuberosity 2*f*, 18*f*, 22, 24*f*
Leukocytosis 165
Ligament
    complete discontinuity of 154
    coracoacromial 2, 2*f*
    coracohumeral 2*f*, 25*f*-27*f*
    fibers, partial discontinuity of 154
    glenohumeral 23*f*
Lipoma 47
    arborescens 134
Little finger
    dorsal aspect of 99
    extensor aspect of 81
Low-grade inflammation, chronic 166

M

Magnetic resonance imaging 33
Malignant transformation 125
Medial elbow pain, differential diagnosis of 52
Median nerve
    compressive neuropathy of 65
    course of 72*f*
    diffuse enlargement of 69*f*
    enlarged 69*f*
    fibrolipomatous hamartoma of 68, 70
    secondary compression of 73
    thickened 66*f*
Metacarpal head 83*f*, 85*f*, 87*f*, 88*f*, 92*f*, 96*f*, 97*f*, 99*f*, 104*f*, 105*f*
    dorsal cortex of 90*f*, 91*f*
Metacarpophalangeal joint
    dorsal aspect of 99*f*
    dorsal recess of 90*f*, 91*f*
    dorsal surface of 81*f*, 99*f*
    ulnar aspect of 104*f*
Metallic implants, position of 40*f*
Microtrauma, recurrent 166
Morel-Lavallée lesions 142, 143
Morel-Lavallée pathophysiology 143*f*
Muscle 34*f*, 142*f*
    adductor group of 106*f*
    enlargement 165
    fascia 116*f*
    fibers 116*f*
        perilesional 41*f*
    hernia 141*f*
    hyperechoic appearance of 165
    retraction 115, 139
    semimembranosus 137*f*
Musculoskeletal ultrasound 90
Mycobacterium leprae 43
Myoaponeurotic junction 56, 56*f*, 117, 130*f*, 138*f*, 139
Myositis ossificans 61, 62
Myotendinous junction, proximal 59*f*

N

Naked cartilage sign 7*f*
Nerve
    distal segment of 40*f*
    fascicles, fat separating 69*f*
    injuries, traumatic 37
    median 63*f*
    traversing elbow 37*f*
Nodular
    calcification 52*f*
    echogenic intratendinous foci 12*f*
    soft tissue calcification 112*f*
    synovial hypertrophy 16*f*
    thickening, focal 89*f*
Nodule
    echogenic 34*f*
    painful 71*f*
    painless 53*f*

O

Olecranon bursitis 44, 44*f*, 45, 45*f*
Osseous avulsion injury 60, 154
    partial-thickness 58
Overuse syndromes 152

P

Pain
    acute 159
    and mild swelling 162
    and stiffness, acute 12
    and swelling, acute 57, 59, 130, 138*f*
    and vague tingling sensation 65
    chronic 15, 132, 144, 147, 164
    focal 89
    intermittent 1
    left elbow 48
    over left knee, chronic 134
Painful erythematous swelling 104, 106, 113
Painless nodules, multiple 63, 63*f*
Painless swelling, intermittent 140
Palmaris longus 63*f*
    tendons 63*f*
Palpable lump, painless 41
Partial-thickness
    articular surface tear 4, 5*f*
    tear 4*f*, 5*f*, 19*f*, 22*f*, 48*f*, 49*f*, 56*f*, 106*f*, 107*f*, 110*f*, 114*f*, 138*f*, 139*f*, 145, 145*f*, 155*f*
        chronic 56, 107
        location of 9
Patella
    anterior cortex of 119*f*
    upper pole of 127
Patellar tendinosis 127
Patellar tendon 126*f*, 128*f*, 131
    focal tendinosis of 127
    full-thickness
        midsubstance tear of 129
        tear of 128, 129
Pennate pattern, loss of 115, 165*f*
Pericapsular crystal deposition disease 87
Peri-insertional fibers, heterogeneous appearance of 52*f*
Peripheral nerve sheath tumor 71, 72
Peritendinitis 145
Peroneal tendons, location of 163*f*
Peroneus brevis tendon 162*f*, 163*f*
    interstitial tear of 162, 163
    invagination of 162*f*
Peroneus longus 162*f*, 163
    tendon 162*f*, 163*f*
Phalanx, middle 81*f*, 82*f*, 92*f*
Pisiform bone 66*f*
Plantar fascia 166, 166*f*, 167
    acute tears of 167
    adjacent 167
    common pathologies of 166
    hypoechoic appearance of 167
    rupture of 166
    thickness 167
Plantar fasciitis 166, 167

Plantar fibromatosis 166
Plantar flexion 149f, 150
Popeye sign 21
Pre-achilles bursitis 153
Prepatellar bursitis 119-121
Proximal forearm, anterior aspect of 59
Proximal patellar tendon, focal inflammation of 126f
Proximal phalanx 81f, 83f, 85f, 87f-90f, 92f, 94f, 96f, 97f, 99f, 104f, 105f
    dorsal cortex of 92f
Psoriasis 152
Pubic symphysis 106f
Puncture wound 36f
Pyomyositis 165

Q

Quadriceps tendon 120f, 125f, 130f, 131
    full-thickness tear of 130
    midsubstance tear of 130f
    retracted 130f
Quadriceps tear 131f

R

Radial artery 64f
Radial nerve 37f
    contusion of 37
    injury 36
    mild thickening of 40f
    stretch injury of 39, 40
    waviness of 40f
Radial styloid 74f
Reactive joint effusion 87
Rectus femoris
    muscle 117f
    partial-thickness tear of 116, 116f
    tendon, partial-thickness tear of 117
Retroachilles bursitis 146f, 152
Retrocalcaneal bursitis 146f, 152, 152f, 153
    causes of 152
Rheumatoid arthritis 24, 53, 54, 73, 85, 89, 90, 120f, 135
Rheumatoid nodule 54
    subcutaneous 53, 54
Road traffic accident 34, 128, 142
Rotator cuff
    calcific tendinosis of 12
    full-thickness tear of 7
    partial-thickness articular surface tear of 4
    subacromial impingement of 1
    tears, morphology of 8f
    tendon 6f

S

Sagging peribursal fat sign 9
Scapula, superior margin of 30f
Schwannomas 72
Semi-liquid calcification 14f
Sesamoid bones 86f
Sessile exostosis 124, 124f, 125
Sharp pain 24, 101, 103
Shoulder
    abduction 1
    anterior aspect of 24
    asymptomatic contralateral 26f
    contralateral asymptomatic 29f
    impingement 2, 3
    joints, bilateral 32f
    pain 4, 10, 25
    paralabral cyst of 30
Simple fluid 136
Skier's thumb 105
Soft swelling, painless 34
Soft tissue
    calcification 55f
        diffuse 157f
        over medial epicondyle 51f
        periarticular 61f
        periarticular amorphous 157f
    echogenic 79f
    hypoechoic 98f, 99f
    peritendinous 161f
Solid hypoechoic lesion 72f
Spinoglenoid notch 29f, 30
Squamous epithelium, proliferation of 82
Subacromial-subdeltoid bursa 2, 5f, 6, 7f, 8f, 12, 14f-16f
Subcutaneous fat 34f, 45f, 53f, 108f, 119f, 142f
Subscapularis tendon 18f
    deep fibers of 1f, 19f
    full-thickness tear of 19
    tear of 18
Subungual glomus tumor 101-103
Superficial infrapatellar bursitis 122, 123f
Suprapatellar recess 132, 134
Suprascapular nerve 30
    course of 30f
    entrapment 29, 30
Suprascapular notch 30f
Supraspinatus tendon 2, 12, 5f, 12f, 27f
    articular surface fibers of 4f
    contralateral 1f
    fibers 5f, 10f
        discontinuity of 7f
    full-thickness retear of 11
    full-thickness tear of 8
    partial-thickness articular surface tear of 4
    posterior fibers of 4f, 8f
    postoperative retear of 10
    recurrent tear of 11f
    tendinosis of 2
Swelling
    in left arm 20
    intermittent 140f
    over
        lateral malleolus 157f
        left knee 132
        posterior aspect of elbow 44
    painful 32, 71, 94, 104f, 122, 138f, 165
    painless 53, 137, 156
Synovial effusion 91
Synovial fluid 91
Synovial hypertrophy 15f, 44f, 78f, 90f, 91, 91f, 94f, 95f, 108f, 118f, 120f, 121, 122f, 132f, 135f, 136
    detection of 24
    mild 46f
Synovial sheath 84
Synovial thickening 73f
    diffuse 73f
Synovitis 135
    acute 118
    inflammatory 90
Synovium
    excised 80f
    hypertrophied 45f
    nodular hypertrophy of 134f
    over extensor tendons, thickened 78f
    thick 136

T

Taenia solium 42
Talofibular ligament, anterior 154, 154f, 155f
Tears
    articular surface 4f, 6, 6f
    complete 139, 155f
    edges of 159f
    extent of 114
    interstitial 144, 144f, 145f, 151, 151f, 159f
    intrasubstance 5f, 6, 6f
    intratendinous 5f
    location of 114
    longitudinal 159f
    margins of 56f, 139f
    partial 127, 139
        thickness 6, 48, 111, 139
    types of 6f
Tendinosis 1f, 2, 5f, 50, 91, 95, 127, 144, 145
    chronic 127
    diffuse 145f
    focal 1f, 2
    insertional 145, 146f

Tendon
- articular surface of 5*f*
- critical zone of 7*f*
- enlargement of 50, 111, 151
- hamstring group of 114*f*
- infraspinatus 12
- sheath 159*f*
    - diffuse thickening of 74*f*, 75*f*
    - giant-cell tumor of 98
    - peroneal 163
- tear 128*f*

Tennis elbow 48
Tennis leg 138, 139
Tenosynovitis 24, 73, 76, 79, 91, 94, 95*f*, 159, 160
- inflammatory 78
- mild 163

Tensor fascia lata 108*f*, 111*f*
Teres minor 2*f*
Thenar eminence 86*f*
Thumb, dorsal aspect of 97, 97*f*
Tibial tuberosity 123*f*
Tibialis anterior muscle
- herniation of 140, 141*f*
- transfascial herniation of 141

Tibialis posterior tendon 159, 160*f*
- inframalleolar segment of 161*f*
- interstitial tear of 159, 160
- location of 160*f*
- retromalleolar segment of 159*f*, 160*f*

Tibiofemoral joint space, medial 134

Tibiofibular ligament, anterior inferior 155*f*
Tibiotalar joint, anterior 154, 154*f*
Tophaceous gout, chronic 156, 158
Torn biceps tendon 21*f*
Torn patellar tendon 129*f*
Trauma 108
Traumatic injuries, evaluation of 38
Triceps muscle 41*f*, 42
- chronic partial-thickness tear of 55
- intramuscular cysticercosis of 41
- medial head of 56, 56*f*

Triceps tendon 45*f*
- osseous avulsion injury of 57
- partial-thickness osseous avulsion injury of 58*f*
- posterior third of 58
- tear 58*f*

Trigger finger 83, 84
Trigger thumb 85
Tubercle, peroneal 163*f*

U

Ulnar artery 66*f*, 73*f*
Ulnar collateral ligament 52, 60*f*, 104*f*
- avulsion injury of 105
- full-thickness tear of anterior band of 60
- injury 104
- normal appearance of 105*f*

of elbow, partial-thickness tears of 60
thickened 104*f*
Ulnar nerve 36*f*, 66*f*
- contusion of 37
- diffuse thickening of 43*f*
- distribution of 43
- injury 36
- neuritis 43

Ulnar neuritis 43
Ulnotrochlear joint space 60

V

Vague pain 55
Vague tingling sensation 68
Valgus strain on elbow 60
Valgus stress 60
Villonodular synovitis, pigmented 47

W

Wooden splinter granuloma 164
Wrist 77*f*
- dorsal
    - and ulnar aspect of 79*f*
    - aspect of 78*f*, 79*f*
- drop 39*f*
- ganglion 63
- radial aspect of 64*f*, 74
- volar aspect of 63, 63*f*, 68, 71, 71*f*

EU GSPR Authorised Reprsentative
Logos Europe, 9 rue Nicolas Poussin
1700, La Rochelle, France
Phone: +33 (0) 6 67 93 73 78
E-mail: contact@logoseurope.eu